The Prescription Drug Problem

The Prescription Drug Problem

A New American Crisis?

Ryan D. Schroeder, Jason A. Ford, and
George E. Higgins

PRAEGER™

An Imprint of ABC-CLIO, LLC
Santa Barbara, California • Denver, Colorado

Library of Congress Cataloging-in-Publication Data

Names: Schroeder, Ryan D., author. | Ford, Jason A., author. | Higgins, George E., author.
Title: The prescription drug problem : a new American crisis? / Ryan D. Schroeder, Jason A. Ford, and George E. Higgins.
Description: Santa Barbara, California : Praeger, [2019] | Includes bibliographical references and index. |
Identifiers: LCCN 2018048752 (print) | LCCN 2018050701 (ebook) | ISBN 9781440857706 (ebook) | ISBN 9781440857690 (cloth : alk. paper)
Subjects: | MESH: Prescription Drug Misuse | Substance-Related Disorders | Health Policy | United States
Classification: LCC RA401.A3 (ebook) | LCC RA401.A3 (print) | NLM WM 270 | DDC 362.29/9—dc23
LC record available at https://lccn.loc.gov/2018048752

ISBN: 978-1-4408-57690 (print)
978-1-4408-57706 (ebook)

23 22 21 20 19 1 2 3 4 5

This book is also available as an eBook.

Praeger
An Imprint of ABC-CLIO, LLC

ABC-CLIO, LLC
147 Castilian Drive
Santa Barbara, California 93117
www.abc-clio.com

This book is printed on acid-free paper ♾

Manufactured in the United States of America

Contents

List of Tables

Introduction

A Prescription for Misuse, Loss, and Destruction

The New American Drug Scare?

The headlines are overwhelming and terrifying: "America's Addiction," "Inside a Killer Drug Epidemic," "Opioids Contribute to a Rising Death Toll," and "Drug Deaths Reach White America" are just a few of the hundreds of stories in the *New York Times* detailing the prescription drug misuse problem in the United States over the past three years. These stories of opioids, destruction, and death have painted a picture of prescription drug misuse sweeping across the nation, exposing every single American to the horrors of addiction. As detailed throughout this book, there is no doubt that prescription drug misuse is a significant problem in the United States, but the headlines and related stories are eerily reminiscent of the headlines associated with the last American drug scare—crack cocaine during the 1980s.

In their 1997 edited collection *Crack in America,* Craig Reinarman and Harry Levine detail the crack cocaine drug scare, including the emergence of the drug and the political and media responses to the problem. In the book, the authors define drug scares as "periods when antidrug crusades have achieved great prominence and legitimacy."[1] Drug scares are essentially campaigns against "demon drugs" that have been used as scapegoats for major social problems such as poverty, crime, violence, broken families, educational failures, and economic decline. The first major drug scare in the United States focused on alcohol and involved middle-class and corporate-elite prohibitionists successfully demonizing the substance as the cause of social problems that surfaced during the rise of American industrialization. In short, the prohibitionist movement was waged against working-class and poor Americans in an effort to control such "unruly" people who were viewed as a threat to the dominant social order of the time.[2]

The elite class's fear of "threatening" populations similarly fueled the other 19th- and 20th-century drug scares. For instance, the first law against opium smoking in the United States was driven at least in part by anti-Chinese sentiments in the 1870s. Chinese immigrants were brought to the United States as laborers to assist in constructing railroads and gold mines during the 19th-century westward American expansion. Opium was the drug of choice for many of the Chinese immigrants, and once the railroad was complete and the gold mines were depleted, the Chinese laborers became an economic threat. Newspapers began running "lurid, fictional newspaper accusations of Chinese men drugging white women into sexual slavery."[3] These newspaper stories were used to generate support among the American population for criminalizing the *smoking* of opium. Note that the other non-Chinese uses of opium, mostly for medicinal purposes, remained legal in the United States at that point. Clearly, the opium smoking crusade was waged as a way to control the Chinese immigrant population.

The first cocaine scare that led to the first federal antidrug law, the 1914 Harrison Act, was also fueled by racial and socioeconomic fears, not in response to any addiction or crime issues. At the dawn of the 20th century, cocaine use had begun shifting from middle- and upper-class whites to the "disreputable" groups of working-class men and black Americans. During this period, the news media once again started publishing salacious and blatantly false stories about cocaine causing African American men to rape white women. David Musto, a medical historian at Yale in the 1970s, showed that the first cocaine scare was clearly racialized, driven by "white alarm" about black Americans rebelling against segregation and oppression.[4]

The criminalization of marijuana was also motivated by racial fears. Marijuana was brought to the United States as the drug of choice by Mexican immigrants, who were brought to the country to fill the labor needs of the railroads, farms, and ranches in the westward U.S. expansion during the late 19th and early 20th centuries. As the Great Depression began and Mexican labor was no longer needed, Harry Anslinger, a former chief of the Federal Bureau of Narcotics, began circulating alarming propaganda to newspapers about the dangers of marijuana, including the claims that marijuana made Mexicans particularly violent. As a result, the marijuana drug scare led the American public to support the 1937 passage of the Marijuana Tax Act, which effectively criminalized the manufacture, possession, and consumption of marijuana. The 1960s witnessed the second marijuana drug scare but in direct opposition to the first marijuana drug scare that portrayed marijuana as leading to violence. The second marijuana scare depicted the drug as creating laziness and un-American sentiments among the 1960s youths who characterized the counterculture that opposed the Vietnam War.

The most recent drug scare revolved around crack cocaine in the 1980s. Cocaine in powder form had been used for decades prior to the crack scare, with use peaking in the late 1970s mainly by affluent white Americans. Wealthy white Americans had even been using cocaine in the powerful and dangerous form of smoking the drug—freebasing—prior to the crack scare. Reinarman and Levine document that the crack scare therefore did not arise out of any substantial increase in the use of cocaine, nor did it arise out of the shift to using the drug in a more direct and dangerous way. Rather, the authors claim that the intense media and political emphasis on crack, beginning in 1986 and persisting until 1992, only developed when cocaine use entered poor, urban minority communities in the form of crack. As Reinarman and Levine state, "politicians and the media focused on crack—and the drug scare began—when cocaine smoking became visible among a 'dangerous' group. Crack attracted the attention of politicians and the media because of its downward mobility to and increased visibility in ghettos and barrios. . . . Crack spread cocaine smoking into poor populations already beset with a cornucopia of troubles."[5] The reasoning provided is that wealthy white cocaine users had a stake in conformity (i.e., jobs) and thus had reason to "cut down, quit, or get private treatment" when their use became problematic. The poorer users of crack, however, "tended to have fewer bonds to conventional society, less to lose and far fewer resources to cope with or shield themselves from drug-related problems."[6] Like prior drug scares, racial fears were part of the reason the crack scare emerged.

The media and political reaction to the appearance of crack in poor urban communities was intense. The first mention of the new form of cocaine was in a 1984 *Los Angeles Times* article, but 1986—a congressional election year—marked the year in which media and political attention to crack skyrocketed. *Time* and *Newsweek* both devoted 5 cover stories each to crack, CBS News ran a documentary on crack that earned the highest television ratings for any similar program in the prior five years, *Time* called crack "the Issue of the Year," and *Newsweek* claimed that crack was the biggest story since the Vietnam War and the Watergate scandal—all in 1986. In a one-year period between 1988 and 1989, the *Washington Post* alone published over 1,500 stories about the crack crisis.[7] In 1988 *ABC News* produced a powerful documentary on the effects of crack, claiming that extensive financial and social damage was the result of crack. "This program did not give its millions of viewers any evidence to support such dramatic claims, but it did give them a powerful *vocabulary of attrition:* 'drugs,' especially crack, threatened all the central institutions in American life—families, communities, schools, businesses, law enforcement, even national sovereignty."[8] A 1989 *New York Times/CBS News* poll showed that 64 percent of Americans believed that drugs were the most important issue facing the country, up from 1 percent of Americans who answered likewise in the same 1985 poll. Clearly, the media attention on crack created a context of fear among the American public.

Politicians across the ideological spectrum responded to the media frenzy surrounding crack—Democrats and Republicans alike campaigned for tough criminal justice drug policies in the 1986 and 1988 elections. Under the guise of the vocabulary of attrition that used crack as a scapegoat for the numerous social ills and failings at the time, Republicans used the crack crisis to push a conservative "tough on crime" agenda, while Democrats used the crack crisis to show that they too were "tough on crime" to win back Democratic defectors. The end result of the intense and often overwhelming media and political attention on crack was the enactment of the War on Drugs, which was originally started during Richard Nixon's presidency but was greatly enhanced and funded during Ronald Reagan's presidency and beyond. The War on Drugs imposed significant punishments on the manufacture, sale, and use of drugs and dramatically increased the budgets for the federal agencies responsible for enforcement of drug laws. For instance, the budget for the Drug Enforcement Administration quadrupled between 1981 and 1992.[9] The crack scare ended by 1992, as media outlets began turning attention to other issues to retain readers and viewers and as politicians became ensnared by the failures of the War on Drugs.

What do the alcohol, marijuana, cocaine, heroin, and crack scares have to do with the current prescription drug misuse crisis in the United States? All of the previous drug scares have included the same basic features. First, prior drug scares have demonized a particular substance associated with a specific racial or ethnic group that was viewed as a threat to the dominant population during a specific historical period. Second, the particular drug has been used as a scapegoat for other major social problems at the time. Third, prior drug scares have resulted in the legal prohibition of the particular substance. Fourth and most important, the extreme reactions to the demonized substances in prior drug scares occurred without any evidence that the drugs in question were being used at an increasing rate or causing any ill effects in society. To illustrate this final point in relation to the latest drug scare over crack, the 1992 National Household Survey on Drug Abuse showed that only 3 percent of 18- to 35-year-olds—the group most likely to use drugs—had "ever used" crack. The same survey showed that less than one-third of those who had ever used crack had used the drug in the prior year.[10] "In short, the evidence indicated that the lifetime prevalence of crack use began low and declined thereafter. And, despite all the claims that it is 'instantaneously addicting,' a clear majority of those who do try it do not continue to use it."[11] Despite the lack of evidence to support the national terror over crack cocaine as well as the other substances that have been demonized in other drug scares, the end result of drug scares is always the same—a criminal justice crackdown on the drugs and drugs users.

Do prescription drugs represent a new American drug scare? This question will be debated throughout the book, but it is important to note a few generalized differences between the prior drug scares and the current problem of prescription drug misuse in the United States. First, prescription drugs remain legal when appropriately prescribed and used. There are in fact legitimate therapeutic uses for the prescription medications, whereas the medical uses of the prior demonized substances are nonexistent (i.e., alcohol and cocaine) or extremely limited (i.e., the use of heroin derivatives or marijuana for pain management). Second, there is no apparent racialized component to the prescription drug misuse crisis. In fact, prescription drug misuse is most often highlighted as a middle-class and/or white predicament, evidenced by OxyContin being termed "hillbilly heroin." Third, as we document in detail in the next chapter, there is evidence that prescription drug misuse has increased at times over the past 20 years. Fourth, the extreme criminal justice response to the current prescription drug misuse problem is missing. As we document later in the book, the criminal justice system has certainly been part of crafting solutions to the prescription drug misuse problem, but the majority of efforts to stem the prescription drug misuse crisis have focused on an element that was notably missing from all of the prior drug scares—public calls for treatment.

All of the notable differences between the current prescription drug misuse crisis and the prior drug scares aside, prescription drug misuse has certainly dominated media and political coverage over the past several years. The *New York Times*, for instance, published over 70 articles on prescription drug misuse in one year alone (July 2016 to July 2017), not to mention the thousands of articles and exposés published by smaller newspapers across the country. Furthermore, prescription drug misuse was a prominent theme of the 2016 presidential and congressional election.

In fact, one of the sticking points in the 2017 congressional debate about health care was whether the federal government would continue to support prescription drug abuse treatment. Therefore, the current prescription drug problem is prominent in the media and politics, and it is possible that the United States is experiencing a new American drug scare. It is equally possible that unlike the previous American drug scares, the prescription drug abuse epidemic is real, verified in the national data and warranting swift and severe public policies.

The Normalization of Drug Abuse

The misuse of pharmaceutical medication is not new or particularly novel. People have been abusing medications provided by medical doctors for over 200 years. Pharmaceutical addiction and misuse, however, was largely hidden and seen as a concern that was limited to a small number of families and contained within the home. But due to the dramatic and sustained rise in the prevalence of prescription drug misuse and the undeniable destructive impact that these addictions have on families and communities, prescription drug misuse has become a major social problem. As we detail throughout the book, prescription drug misuse has destroyed countless lives, families, and communities. Communities can no longer ignore the prescription drug misuse problem or relegate prescription drug misuse as a private family concern. Prescription drug misuse is a deadly and destructive problem that affects everybody.

The primary factor that distinguishes prescription drug misuse from the use of other illicit drugs (i.e., cocaine, heroin, methamphetamine) is that prescription drug misuse has been normalized. To illustrate the normalization of prescription drug misuse, the first author of this book begins his prescription drug misuse lecture with a fictitious story about having stayed up all night working on the lecture. He then explains that he used Adderall given to him by a friend to help him complete the lecture. The reaction by the students to the admission that a prescription medication was misused to complete a lecture is always the same—no reaction. The first author of the book then changes the story to include the use of methamphetamine to help him stay awake and complete the lecture, to which the students react with overwhelming shock and disgust. The first author then asks the students to explain why they react differently to the admission of methamphetamine to complete the lecture than to the admission of Adderall to complete the lecture. After all, as the first author explains to his student, Adderall and methamphetamine are both classified as stimulants and work to achieve the same goal of staying awake to complete the lecture. This generates a lively classroom discussion in which students attempt to justify, neutralize, and normalize the misuse of prescription medications and stigmatize the use of other illicit drugs. This classroom exercise is designed to show that prescription medications are perceived as safe, legitimate, and used by respectable people but that illicit drugs are dangerous, stigmatized, and used only by disreputable people. Perhaps the normalization of prescription drug misuse is the most important—and dangerous—factor behind the dramatic rise in and the deadly consequences of prescription drug misuse.

Contrary to popular perceptions evidenced by the reaction of students in the classroom exercise described above, prescription medications are drugs. As defined by the U.S. government in Title 21 United States Code Controlled Substances Act (321(g)(1)), "The term 'drug' means (A) articles recognized in the official United States Pharmacopoeia, official Homeopathic Pharmacopoeia of the United States, or official National Formulary, or any supplement of any of them; and (B) articles intended for use in the diagnosis, cure, mitigation, treatment, or prevention of disease in man or other animals; and (C) articles (other than food) intended to affect the structure or any function of the body of man or other animals; and (D) articles intended for use as a component of any article specified in clause (A), (B), or (C)." Similar to other illicit drugs such as heroin, cocaine, methamphetamine, and marijuana, prescription drugs are also considered controlled substances (Schedules I–V) defined in the same law (821(b)(2–5)). Just as the use or possession of other illicit drugs is a violation of the law and is subject to criminal penalty, using a prescription medication in a manner other than prescribed, using a prescription medication that was not prescribed to the individual, and/or possessing a prescription medication without a valid prescription are also clear violations of the Controlled Substances Act and subject to criminal penalties outlined in the law. In short, U.S. law treats prescription medication as any other illicit drugs when used or possessed in any way outside the provisions of the prescription. Prescription drug misuse is drug use.

Despite the relative normalization of prescription drug misuse in the United States, the dangers and consequences of prescription drug misuse are gradually emerging in media representations and public discourse. In this chapter, we highlight many of the high-profile prescription drug use tragedies that have elevated the problems of prescription drug misuse into the national spotlight. We then share case studies of individuals and communities ravaged by prescription drug misuse and addiction. The stories of celebrities who have died from prescription drug overdoses, individuals battling prescription drug addiction, and the specific communities destroyed by the prescription drug epidemic personalize the prescription drug misuse problem that is pervasive in the United States. The last section of the chapter provides basic information needed to understand alarming nationwide trends in prescription drug misuse, a brief history of prescription drug misuse in the United States, definitions of prescription drugs that are prone to misuse that will be examined throughout the rest of the book, and a description of the differences between prescription drug misuse and the use of other illicit drugs.

Famous, Addicted, and Dead

The routinization of caricature—when the worst cases are portrayed as the typical cases in the media and dominant cultural narrative—is central to discussions of drug use trends in the United States. The crack epidemic, for instance, was characterized by Len Bias, a star basketball player at the University of Maryland who was drafted by the Boston Celtics as the second overall pick in the 1986 National Basketball Association draft. Bias died two days after the draft following a night of partying with his college teammates. The cause of Bias's death was cardiac arrhythmia caused by cocaine use,[12] possibly in the form of crack.[13] Just eight days later another famous athlete, Don Rogers, a football star at the University of California–Los Angeles and a safety for the Cleveland Browns in the National Football League, was found dead of a cocaine overdose,[14] again possibly in the form of crack. The apparent crack-related deaths of these two famous, privileged athletes were largely responsible for the explosion in media and political coverage of the drug crisis generally and the crack epidemic specifically.

The prescription drug misuse problem has not been immune to the routinization of caricature. In fact, the routinization of caricature associated with the prescription drug problem has been more intense and has occurred over a much longer period of time than prior drug epidemics. Celebrities have long been featured as prescription drug addicts, and there is no shortage of heavily covered celebrity tragedies associated with prescription drug misuse.

The death of the musician Prince on April 21, 2016, at the age of 57 brought the serious and deadly problem of prescription drug misuse to the national spotlight. Prince was found unresponsive inside an elevator in his home in Chanhassen, Minnesota, with prescription opioids in his possession. Although full autopsy and toxicology reports were not released to the public, the medical examiner's office reported that the cause of Prince's death was "the decedent self-administered fentanyl" and defined his death as "accidental."[15] Fentanyl is a powerful prescription opioid medication typically prescribed to cancer patients that is hundreds of times more potent than heroin.[16]

But Prince reportedly struggled with opioid addiction for several years prior to his overdose death. According to news reports taken from his half siblings, Prince was addicted to Percocet, another prescription opioid medication, for decades prior to his death. Similar to most stories of prescription drug misuse told throughout the book, Prince's addiction to opioids began as a way to medically manage the tolls of touring and performing, not for recreational use, but his medical use of Percocet eventually developed into misuse, addiction, and death.

Less than a week before he was found dead, Prince's plane made an emergency landing in Moline, Illinois, on his return trip to Minnesota after a performance in Atlanta. Prince was found unresponsive in the plane and was rushed to a local hospital, where he was treated for a prescription drug overdose. Prince's addiction was so severe that the day before he died, his team called an opioid addiction specialist, Dr. Howard Kornfeld, for immediate help. The situation was described as a "grave medical emergency" by Prince's attorney.[17] Dr. Kornfeld could not get to Minnesota immediately, so he sent his son Andrew on an overnight flight to immediately evaluate Prince's health, encourage him to enter treatment for his prescription opioid addiction, and possibly administer a medication, buprenorphine, used to treat opioid addiction. The goal was to bring Prince to California for long-term addiction treatment. But Andrew Kornfeld arrived too late to save Prince's life. Andrew, along with two of Prince's representatives, found Prince dead, full of fentanyl, with even more prescription opioids in his possession. His death was an accident, not a suicide, fueled by an uncontrollable addiction. Prince was yet another tragic victim of prescription drug misuse.

Upon his death, Prince was added to the long and growing list of celebrities who have died from a prescription drug overdose or from the combination of prescription drug misuse and alcohol or other illicit drug use. Heath Ledger, who was famous for his high-profile acting roles including as the Joker in the *Dark Knight,* among other popular and award-winning films, died on January 22, 2008, at the age of 28. The New York City medical examiner concluded that "Mr. Ledger died as the result of acute intoxication by the combined effects of oxycodone, hydrocodone, diazepam, temazepam, alprazolam, and doxylamine."[18] Although these different prescription medications will be explained in more detail later, the lethal cocktail of medications that killed Ledger included narcotic painkillers, antianxiety drugs, and sleep medications. His death was also deemed accidental, not a suicide, and it appears that he was prescribed the medications to treat pneumonia and sleeplessness. But some reporting suggests that Ledger was addicted to sleeping medications[19] along with a variety of other drugs.

Prescription drugs also tragically took the life of Michael Jackson, the world-famous "King of Pop." Jackson was a well-known prescription drug addict, having cancelled his 1993 *Dangerous* tour to seek treatment for prescription pain killer abuse.[20] Demerol, Percocet, and Darvocet, all prescription opioid medications that were prescribed to Jackson following injuries sustained from a fire in 1984 as well as numerous cosmetic surgeries throughout his life, sparked Jackson's decades of prescription opioid misuse.[21] During the 1993 tour Jackson's wife, Debbie Rowe, reported that he had become a "hot mess" and pushed him to seek addiction treatment.[22] After years of prescription drug misuse, Jackson was found in bed not breathing on June 25, 2009.

Although Jackson struggled with his addiction to prescription opioids for decades, his death was caused by another prescription medication—propofol. Propofol is a surgical anesthetic that was repeatedly administered by Dr. Conrad Murray to help Jackson sleep. Jackson's autopsy report concluded that his death was an "acute propofol intoxication" along with numerous other prescription sedative medications.[23] Dr. Murray was eventually convicted of involuntary manslaughter and sentenced to four years in prison for his improper administering of propofol to Jackson.

Bruce Lee, the famous martial arts actor, also died from a complication associated with a prescription pain reliever and anxiety medication, Equagesic, that was given to him by a friend.[24] Anna Nicole Smith, a model and actress, was killed by a lethal cocktail of nine prescription medications, mostly antianxiety drugs, on February 8, 2007. Although the medications were prescribed to Smith and taken as prescribed, the interaction of the medications led to her accidental overdose death. Similarly, Brittany Murphy, an actress, died on December 24, 2009, with elevated levels of prescription hydrocodone, among a variety of other over-the-counter and prescription medications, in her body. Controversy continues to surround Murphy's death, but in an interview with *CBS News* in 2009 a medical doctor stated,

> When you have a 32-year-old person dying suddenly, and especially a celebrity in Los Angeles, you can place your bet down that it's going prove to be a case of acute combined drug toxicity. And I bet you that this young lady tragically died in the same way that Michael Jackson did, and Anna Nicole Smith, and her son, Daniel Smith, and Heath Ledger—a combination of

> drugs that had been prescribed for her, prescribed for her husband, for her mother, in some fictitious names, probably by doctors who are very, very quick to make available anything that celebrities want, sometimes using knowingly fictitious names. . . . So, even though these drugs are, quote, legal, unquote, they are, many times, illegally obtained. And it's a tragedy. And it's being played out everywhere in America every day, and we only come to know about it when it involves celebrities.[25]

Perhaps the celebrity poster child of prescription drug misuse, a term expressed by California's attorney general Jerry Brown, was Cory Haim, the star of dozens of movies including *The Lost Boys*. Haim had abused prescription medications for more than 20 years and had been in and out of drug treatment facilities most of his life. He died after collapsing in his home on March 10, 2010.[26] Although Haim's final autopsy report claimed that he died from an enlarged heart and narrowing blood vessels not specifically linked to his well-known drug addiction, and although the death was ruled "natural," subsequent investigations revealed that Haim had been doctor shopping—visiting multiple doctors over a short period of time for the express purpose of obtaining numerous prescriptions—for months before his death. He had obtained at least 533 powerful prescription pills, including opioid painkillers, shortly before his death, and investigators found several prescription medication bottles in his bedroom.[27] Prescription drug misuse ravaged Haim's life and likely contributed in some part to his tragic and untimely death.

Even Whitney Houston's death on February 11, 2012, has been attributed, at least partially, to prescription drug misuse. The Grammy Award–winning singer had a long history of drug use, including cocaine and prescription drug misuse. Although the official autopsy revealed that Houston's death was an accidental drowning with artery blockage and cocaine use as contributing factors, investigators found numerous prescription medications, mainly antianxiety drugs including Xanex and Flexeril (a prescription muscle relaxer), in the hotel room where Houston died.[28] An *ABC News* report in 2012 quotes Dr. Cyril Wecht, a forensic pathologist, as stating that Houston's drowning was likely influenced by taking numerous prescription medications that caused her to not wake up after her head went under the water in the bathtub: "If you are deeply unconscious to the point of a deep stupor, then it is conceivable that there was a heavy concentration of drugs."[29] Because Houston had a long history of cocaine and alcohol misuse, it is possible that her prescription drug problem developed during her many rehabilitation attempts. In the same *ABC News* report, Alesandra Rain, cofounder of a prescription drug rehabilitation program, stated, "What often happens with illegal drug addiction is that the treatment involves legal drugs, which can be even more challenging to quit. . . . Because Xanax is legal, it gives much the false sense that they are safe." It is likely that Houston's attempt to break her addictions to illegal drugs led to her becoming dependent on prescription drugs, which quite possibly contributed to her untimely death.

Similarly, Keith Moon, the drummer for the band the Who, died from an overdose of a prescription sedative, Heminevrin, that he was prescribed to alleviate alcohol withdrawal symptoms. After experiencing a terrible recording session, a movie screening, and a fight with his girlfriend while trying to remain sober, Moon took 32 Heminevrin tablets. He was found dead in his bed by his girlfriend on September 7, 1978, at the age of 32.[30] The coroner found the pills in Moon's stomach, 26 of which were undigested, and concluded that the 6 digested pills were more than enough to kill him. The coroner could not determine whether Moon's death was a suicide or an accident, but those who were close to Moon strongly reject the possibility of suicide. "He loved life too much," his friend and bassist for the Who told *Rolling Stone* magazine shortly after Moon's death. Keith Moon lived a life famous for excess in all realms, and like so many public figures before and after, his life was tragically cut short because of prescription drug misuse.

There is no doubt that the rigors of show business create pressures to cope with substance use, often in the form of nonmedical prescription drug use. Judy Garland, famous for her role as Dorothy in the *Wizard of Oz*, also struggled mightily with prescription pill addiction and misuse throughout her career. By the time Garland was 18 and already a movie star, she was seeing a psychiatrist to help with the stresses of her career. It was then that she started abusing prescription drugs. In the *New York Times* article announcing her death in 1969, Garland was quoted as having stated, "They'd give us pep pills. Then they'd take us to the studio hospital and knock us cold with sleeping pills . . . after four hours, they'd wake us up and give us the pep pills again."[31] Garland's addiction to pills followed her through numerous failed marriages and attempts to resurrect her career. Ultimately, her addiction to prescription medications took her life. Judy Garland was found dead in her London home on June 22, 1969. The official cause of death was "an incautious self-overdosage" of barbiturates.[32] Her death was ruled accidental, yet another tragic reminder of the deadly consequences of prescription drug misuse.

Addiction to prescription pills also claimed the life of Dana Plato, one of the stars of the television series *Diff'rent Strokes*. Plato's life was dominated by addiction to alcohol and other drugs, including prescription opioids. Years of prescription drug misuse led to her death on May 8, 1999. Plato died from an overdose of Lortab, an opioid prescription pain reliever, and Soma, a prescription muscle relaxer. Although Plato's death was officially ruled a suicide, her former manager Gerald Wolff stated shortly after her death that "In my heart of hearts I do not believe she committed suicide. . . . Dana loved life too much."[33]

Marilyn Monroe, the famous model and actress, suffered a similar fate. The long days and stresses of Hollywood caused her to seek out prescription barbiturates, amphetamines, and opioids to help her manage the workload. Monroe reportedly misused these prescription medications for most of her short life.[34] On August 5, 1962, Monroe was found dead in her bedroom, like so many of the celebrities who died from prescription drug overdoses before and after her. The official autopsy report lists the cause of her death as suicide by acute barbiturate poisoning.[35] Controversy surrounded this conclusion, and an investigation into Monroe's cause of the death was opened in 1982, but this investigation came to the same conclusion: that she committed suicide by ingesting an entire bottle of Nembutal, which is a prescription barbiturate. Regardless of whether Monroe's death was accidental or intentional, she was yet another celebrity who met an early death at the hands of prescription drug misuse.

Even Elvis Presley, the world-famous musician, struggled with prescription drug addiction. In a *People* magazine interview in 2016, his stepbrother revealed that Elvis's life was dominated by prescription drug misuse. His stepbrother reported that Elvis maintained "attack packs" of 6 to 11 pills, mainly barbiturates, opioid pain medications, and stimulants, that he would take up to three times per day with one to three shots of Demerol—another opioid painkiller.[36] Elvis's prescription drug misuse was so significant that his stepbrother claimed, "Whomever was watching him had to make sure that the drugs didn't kick in before he was done eating and put him to sleep, or else he risked choking to death, of which he had a couple close calls." Although Elvis's official cause of death was cardiac arrhythmia, an irregular heartbeat, significant controversy surrounds his death to this date.[37] As Guralnick wrote in his 1999 book *Careless Love: The Unmaking of Elvis Presley*, "Drug use was heavily implicated." A lab report conducted following Elvis's death revealed that use of multiple prescription drugs caused his death, as 10 drugs were found in his blood in significant, probably lethal, quantities.[38] Prescription drug misuse certainly characterized Elvis's last years and possibly contributed to his death either directly or indirectly.

The stories of prescription drug misuse, the destruction that their addictions created, and the untimely deaths of these celebrities, along with the numerous other celebrities not included above, stimulated a great deal of media coverage. Celebrity struggles with prescription drug misuse, along with the resulting deaths, are certainly newsworthy and have stimulated limited coverage of the wider prescription drug misuse and addiction problem in our current culture. The stories of celebrities who have struggled with prescription drug misuse are not limited to the celebrity lifestyle—the stories of death and destruction caused by prescription drug misuse are all too common and increasingly prevalent in families across the United States. Prescription drug misuse affects a wide swath of the American public—the wealthy and the homeless, men and women, doctors and nurses, traditional drug users and respectable middle-class professionals. Nobody is immune from the problem of prescription drug misuse. The following section highlights the stories of ordinary Americans who have struggled with and even died from this drug use epidemic that is raging across the country. Their stories are dire and tragic, not much different from the stories of celebrities. But the stories from ordinary Americans also provide glimpses of hope and recovery.

Everyday Struggles with Prescription Drug Misuse and Addiction

One of the defining features that fueled the crack scare was the sensationalized media focus on crack entering middle-class communities. A 1986 *Newsweek* article, for instance, claimed that crack "has transformed the ghetto" and "is rapidly spreading into the suburbs." Other media outlets such as the *New York Times* and *Time* featured stories about the crack plague having spread to middle-class Americans and claiming that the crack epidemic had become "universal"—again, without any evidence.[39]

The prescription drug misuse epidemic was brought to the national spotlight by high-profile celebrity tragedies, much like the crack crisis of the 1980s. But unlike the crack epidemic of the 1980s, the stories of these celebrities who struggled mightily with prescription drug misuse and eventually died, at least in part, from prescription addictions can be told by hundreds of thousands of Americans and their families every year. Newspapers, magazines, and televised news programs have shared many stories of ordinary, often middle-class Americans battling prescription drug misuse over the past two decades. Like the stories from celebrities, the prescription drug misuse stories of ordinary Americans are also dire and often tragic. However, unlike many of the stories from celebrities, whose misuse of prescription medications was largely unknown to the public until it was too late, the stories of ordinary Americans who are addicted to prescription drugs occasionally offer uplifting messages of resolve and recovery.

The Courier-Journal, the local newspaper in Louisville, Kentucky, began a series of articles on the prescription drug misuse problem in 2011. The articles in the series addressed all aspects of the prescription drug misuse epidemic in Kentucky, including so-called pill mills and the interstate distribution of illegal prescriptions, all of which will be addressed in detail later in this book. But the series also focused on numerous Kentucky residents and their families as they dealt with the pains, struggles, and tragic outcomes of prescription drug addictions.

One story was of T. J. Walden. T. J. was generally a good child who came from a military family and joined the national guard after graduating from a prestigious private high school. His mother reported that he did not drink much alcohol as a teenager and only experimented with marijuana a couple of times. But as T. J. neared the end of high school he was introduced to OxyContin, a prescription opioid painkiller, by his friends. Eventually T. J. moved on to misuse Opana, an even more powerful opioid painkiller. His mother reported that his behavior changed when he started abusing prescription opioids: "I knew something was wrong. His behavior had changed. . . . He didn't sleep much at night."[40] T. J. even stole money from his mother. Knowing that something was wrong with T. J., his mother started drug testing him, and he was respectful and honest with his family throughout his addiction. At one point T. J. confided in his mother, "Mom, I don't want to die from this."[41]

T. J. even went through a 30-day recovery program, which his mother paid $11,000 for on a credit card, and he stayed clean for a few months afterward. T. J. was committed to staying sober for his National Guard training, which he completed, and was scheduled to deploy to Africa. Before his deployment, he went camping with his friends. The next day on the morning of July 1, 2012, T. J.'s family was greeted by a police officer who informed them that T. J. was dead from an apparent Opana overdose. T. J.'s mother has become deeply involved in prescription drug misuse prevention efforts. A little more than four years after T. J.'s death his mother stated, "I am not going away. The mistakes that were made need to be corrected. How many people have to die? . . . My son T. J. . . . would have given his life to protect and serve, and he was one of the most patriotic young men. And his country failed him."[42]

T. J.'s pathway to prescription drug addiction—and eventually death—is all too common. One of the recurring themes with prescription drug misuse, and possibly one of the reasons that prescription drug misuse has received so much more attention than most prior drug use epidemics, is that prescription drug addicts such as T. J. tend to come from middle-class families, do well in school, and even hold respected or prestigious jobs. Stated differently, prescription drug misusers do not fit the stereotypical image of drug addicts. Regardless of the way in which these people were introduced to addictive medications, the message sent by T. J.'s mom resonates throughout almost every story—"his country failed him."

The website www.medicineabuseproject.com presents hundreds of stories about prescription drug misuse from ordinary Americans. The stories describe the ways in which the addictions ravaged individual lives and destroyed families but also how recovery and rebuilding are possible. Miss Kentucky Teen USA in 2009, Jefra Bland, in a video on the website, told of her father's addiction to prescription medications during her life. His addiction led to the loss of his successful business, and the family was constantly terrified that he was going to overdose. Bland also recounted his multiple attempts at recovery and his eventual sobriety.

Another post on the website shares "Mark's Story." As written by his father, Mark had a happy childhood, had many friends, played sports, and was active in his church. His parents were completely devoted to Mark and his brother. Although Mark had occasionally experimented with marijuana and beer, his father wrote that "I never associated 'addiction' or 'substance abuse' with my son. In my mind, those were linked to other people from other neighborhoods. I thought of us as the stereotypical middle class family. Substance use was just something I heard about on the news or read about in the newspaper. Unfortunately, I know now that it was also in our own house." After a special day at school, Mark came home, had dinner with his family, lifted weights, and went to work. The next day, Mark was found dead in his bed with a bag of loose prescription pills next to him. The medications were not prescribed to Mark or anybody else in the family. Mark died from an accidental overdose of prescription opioids and amphetamines. No alcohol or other illicit drugs were found in his body. His father wrote, "How could I have let this happen? After all, I had always considered myself a good dad (a great dad, actually). I have always loved my children. We spent time together, read stories, played, etc. . . . Our kids seemingly 'had it made.'" As with many other families destroyed by prescription drug misuse, Mark's father has become involved in outreach efforts to help others avoid the same fate: "I miss my son more than words can express, and life is not the same anymore. I want other parents to learn from me."[43]

Similarly, another mother shared the story of her son, Kent. Like so many stories of prescription drug misuse, Kent was raised in a loving home, was a good student and a Boy Scout, and went to church with his family. He was a normal child from a strong family. But after a night away from his house, Kent's parents discovered that he had been abusing prescription medications and immediately began intervention efforts. His mother wrote, "He did not want to be a drug addict, and after some time, it seemed like he made it out. . . . I thought we were in the clear." After recovery appeared to be a reality for Kent, he had his wisdom teeth removed. As is normal following oral surgery, the dentist gave him a prescription for a painkiller, which his mother had filled and put in the medicine cabinet. After realizing that the bottle was missing pills a few days later, she confronted her son, who admitted to taking some of the medication, and asked him why he wanted to take the pills. His mother reported, "He asked me to remember a time that I felt 'GREAT'—'the best.' When I had the memory, he said, 'the first time you get high—it's BETTER than that. . . . All you can think about is feeling that way again—only it's physically, chemically impossible.'"[44] After this incident, Kent again regained his sobriety and appeared again to have moved on from his prescription drug misuse—he had moved into a house with a couple of roommates, was finishing his first year of college, had a job, and was living independently. But on a Monday morning in September, the family received the feared knock on the door. Kent was dead from a prescription opioid overdose. Another promising life was lost to prescription drugs, another family destroyed.

Describing the aftermath of Kent's tragic death, his mother wrote, "I wish I had been better educated about drugs. . . . Maybe Kent would be alive today. But he isn't. And I live with the pain every day. I'll never get to see him grow up, get married or have children. I'll never see him live his life and realize his dreams. I could spend the rest of my life being angry, but I'm not sure who I should be angry with. I was a good mom! I put a lot of time into my children. And I forgive my son. I'm trying to honor his memory by helping other parents and kids understand the dangers of using drugs—especially prescription drugs. . . . I'm hoping that by telling Kent's story perhaps, just one person will make a different choice."[45]

Aaron was another high achiever whom nobody would have expected to have a raging addiction to prescription drugs. According to the account posted by his sister, Aaron owned a beautiful home in California and had a good job and a loving family. He was a star athlete in high school, but by the time he was in his early 30s, he experienced a great deal of physical pain from the various injuries he sustained through high school sports. The doctor prescribed Vicodin, a prescription opioid drug, to manage the pain, which started a rapid descent into uncontrollable addiction. His sister wrote, "Unlike a lot of addicts, my brother only survived his addiction for about three years. I know that he had hated what he had become and desperately wanted to change. He tried several times to get clean. He even secretly went to rehab at one point but still couldn't beat his addiction to pain pills. My brother was the strongest person I have ever known, which made me realize that addiction has nothing to do with a person's character or strength. I have also realized that addiction has no prejudice!"[46] Aaron's parents found him dead at the age of 36. He had lost his battle with addiction to prescription opioid pills. Describing the grief that followed Aaron's death, his sister wrote, "It has been over three years since he left us, but I still cry every day. My parents and I have tried to move on with our lives because we know this is what Aaron would want, but, honestly, moving on seems like an impossible task some days. Aaron was our sunshine. He was kind and beautiful. I miss him every day of my life. I can no longer call him for advice; I can no longer hear his amazing laugh. I have to live the rest of my life without my best friend."[47] Aaron had quickly become another unlikely victim of prescription drug misuse and left behind a loving family struggling to pick up the pieces of a life destroyed by addiction.

As these cases illustrate, prescription drug misuse has destroyed countless lives. The damage from prescription drug misuse is not limited to the high-profile stories of famous people; rather, the destructive impact of prescription drug misuse is being felt by everyday American citizens—doctors, nurses, teachers, businesspeople, teenagers, and the elderly. No group has been spared from the dirge of prescription drug addiction, misuse, and death. The hopes and dreams of individuals and families are being destroyed by prescription drug misuse every single day in the United States. But are these stories of everyday Americans who struggle with prescription drug misuse and addiction further promoting the routinization of caricature? Or are these stories, combined with the stories of celebrities who have struggled with prescription drug misuse, actually representative of the true prescription drug misuse problem in the United States? A look at specific communities that have been devastated by prescription drug misuse helps shed some light on the true nature of the problem.

Communities Destroyed by Prescription Drug Misuse

Not surprisingly, the problem of prescription drug misuse that continues to devastate individual lives and families is also impacting entire communities. In short, the fabric of American life is being threatened by the deadly and growing epidemic of prescription drug misuse.

The ravages of prescription drug misuse can be seen everywhere in the United States, but no area of the country has been hit harder by the prescription epidemic than Appalachia. This area was the center of the coal mining industry, and as the coal mining industry collapsed in the second half of the 20th century, Appalachia was left with an aging population of former manual laborers struggling with the ailments associated with decades of physical work and a growing population of bored young people with few prospects for a better future. The combination of high rates of prescribed medications, especially prescription opioid painkillers, and a bored and disaffected population of young people created a context that was ripe for widespread prescription drug misuse. And this widespread prescription drug misuse has devastated countless communities in its path.

Sean Dunne's documentary *Oxyana,* for instance, details the devastating effect that prescription drug misuse has had on Oceana, a small coal mining town in West Virginia.[48] The documentary describes in vivid detail the rapid decline of the once thriving classic American rural community. Outsiders would be inclined to view Oceana—filled with natural mountainous beauty, a kind and generous population, and a rich history—as the perfect American town. But prescription drugs, primarily the opioid painkiller OxyContin, quickly infested the community, and the town that was once full of children riding bikes in the streets, where nobody locked their doors, rapidly devolved into a community plagued by addiction, crime, corruption, and prostitution. Death, addiction, and destruction now characterize this small American town.

The tragic and devastating story of the decline of Oceana highlights an all too common problem facing American communities from coast to coast, encompassing both urban and rural areas. In many ways, Oceana is representative of the prescription drug misuse epidemic that is sweeping across the nation and destroying communities in the path of the prescription drug addiction storm. As the film illustrates, OxyContin was introduced into Oceana in the mid-1990s and was heavily marketed to medical doctors as the answer to the chronic pain among the aging coal miners in the town, whose bodies had been ravaged by decades of manual labor. But those pills eventually diffused throughout the entire population of the town. A decline in coal mining jobs and a distressed economy, combined with a population of bored small-town youths, created an intense need for escape in Oceana. The town was quickly overrun with prescription pill addicts and an economy that offered few employment opportunities outside of dealing prescription drugs.

Oceana was destroyed by prescription drug misuse. As one person in the documentary indicated, "I'm 23. Half of my graduating class is dead."

Characterizing the economic conditions of Oceana, another person featured in the documentary stated that "you either work in the mines or you sell pills." Drug treatment centers are overwhelmed, babies are born addicted to prescription medication at a high rate, crime and violence have been normalized, and overdose deaths have skyrocketed in Oceana. And the prospects for improved conditions in Oceana are bleak. Like so many other cities and towns in the United States, the once thriving community has been rendered lifeless at the hands of a powerful and seemingly endless prescription drug scourge.

Kermit, West Virginia, is another small town that has been impacted by prescription drug misuse. Kermit is generally believed to be ground zero for the prescription drug epidemic, not necessarily because the population is addicted to prescription drugs but because a pharmacy in Kermit was filling millions of prescriptions for opioid painkillers. The pharmacy, located in a town of fewer than 400 people, was shipped 9 million opioid painkiller pills over a two-year period. As quoted in an article published by CBS, "They filled more scripts for oxycodone than all but 21 pharmacies in America."[49] Not surprisingly, the county in which Kermit is located has one of the highest rates of prescription drug overdose in the United States. But Kermit was also inundated with other problems associated with the prescription drug misuse problem. As a city council member stated in a *West Virginia Gazette* story, "The entire town was constantly clogged with traffic. You couldn't find a place to park at the post office. It wasn't a safe place to be. They'd come by the vanload. They'd park a van and eight people would get out."[50] Another council member stated, "I was afraid to get out of my vehicle."

Kermit, West, Virginia was an unassuming, friendly, safe small town. But an unscrupulous pharmacist became a kingpin for the prescription drug problem raging across America, and through his actions prescription drug misuse ruined the safety, sanctity, and health of the town. Lawsuits have been filed against the pharmacist and drug distribution companies. Residents hope that removing the bad actors from their town will help Kermit heal from the destructive effects of prescription drug misuse.

War, West Virginia, is another small town in Appalachia plagued by the prescription drug misuse epidemic. A wide-reaching exposé on prescription drug misuse published in *Playboy* magazine in 2014 details the sordid story of War, the mayor, his son, and his daughter-in-law. Like so many stories of small towns destroyed by prescription drug misuse, War was a lively, thriving, scenic mountainous coal-mining town in the 1940s and 1950s. But the combination of the increased mechanization of coal mining and the simultaneous loss of coal mining jobs left War in ruins.

The overdose death rate in McDowell County, where War sits, is currently 16 times higher than the national average. The reporter describes the current state of War:

> Things have gotten worse. War has shrunk to around 1,000 people, one quarter of its peak. The few blocks of low brick buildings that compose War's downtown are a glum procession of empty storefronts, broken windows and a caved-in roof, interspersed with a handful of surviving businesses—including no fewer than three pharmacies. On a window of the War Hotel, the town flophouse, the owners have taped a handwritten sign: NO ALCOHOL OR DRUGS ALLOWED IN THE BUILDING OF ANY KIND. ALL WHO GET COUGHT (sic) WILL GO TO JAIL.
>
> Today, McDowell County is at the bottom of the heap by just about every measure of misery and dysfunction. One third of its inhabitants live below the poverty line. Barely six percent have college degrees. Life expectancy is among the lowest in the nation. The county also has the state's highest rates of teen pregnancy and child abuse.[51]

Tom Hatcher was elected mayor of War in 1997 on a simple platform to bring a water treatment plant, a playground, and a drug treatment facility to the town. He also taught at the high school in War. But it wasn't long before the prescription drug misuse epidemic took its grip on the town and his own family. Hatcher's son had developed an intense addiction to prescription opioids as a teenager in War, influenced by his friends and the prescription drug misuse culture in the town. As Hatcher was trying to address the prescription drug problem in War, he was also trying to address the addiction problem in his own home. He had kept a list of the residents in War who had died from prescription drug overdoses that included dozens of people in just a few years. After years of fighting the prescription drug epidemic in his town and his own home, Hatcher was found dead in his home, apparently killed by his daughter-in-law who was addicted to prescription pills. War has become another victim of the prescription drug misuse epidemic.

Although slightly outside of Appalachia, Chillicothe, Ohio, has also been hit hard by prescription drug misuse. Chillicothe is somewhat different than many of the communities in Appalachia that have been destroyed by prescription drug use, as the city has not been dramatically affected by the decline of the coal industry or deindustrialization more generally. Chillicothe has several major employers, including a hospital, a truck factory, a major paper mill, two prisons, and a branch campus of Ohio University. In other words, good jobs are not difficult to find in Chillicothe. As one resident stated about Chillicothe, "It used to be so

Mayberry."[52] With about 77,000 people, Chillicothe was by all accounts another typical midwestern American town. But the prescription drug epidemic has fundamentally changed the community. A police detective in Chillicothe stated, "Within the last 10 years it's changed significantly. The violent crime rate has gone up, the theft issues have gone up, all driven by the drug issue."[53] The general consensus in Chillicothe is that the prescription drug problem was caused by the city being on "the 23 pipeline," a reference to Highway 23 that has become a primary transportation path for drugs coming from the Ohio River to Columbus, Ohio, and Detroit, Michigan. In this relatively small American town, 40 people died of prescription drug overdoses in 2015.

Far from Appalachia, Everett, Washington, has also been destroyed by prescription drug misuse. Everett, a city of about 100,000 people located between Seattle and the Canadian border, has several large employers, including Boeing and the U.S. Navy. Although the town had struggled with methamphetamine addiction in the past, Everett's most pressing problem today is OxyContin misuse. Gangs organized with rogue doctors and pharmacies in the Los Angeles area to flood Everett with OxyContin that was driven up the Interstate 5 corridor. The opioid-based painkiller spread like a virus through the community, destroying uncountable numbers of lives in its path. As reported by the *Los Angeles Times*,

> Dealers sold pills in parks, outside grocery stores and at car washes. The aluminum foil that addicts used to smoke the pills littered parking lots and sidewalks. Some grocery stores gave away foil squares to discourage the rampant shoplifting of Reynolds Wrap.
>
> Addicts burglarized homes, picked pockets, stole identities, robbed businesses and prostituted themselves. Young women in pasties and thongs offered sexual favors alongside lattes at a proliferation of drive-in "bikini" espresso stands.[54]

Importantly, the article details that OxyContin addiction attracted people who ordinarily would not be considered druggies—"people with no criminal records and stable homes, jobs, and families."[55] OxyContin had infiltrated the homes and lives of middle-class people in Everett, causing the all too common trail of death, devastation, and destruction in the lives of middle-class addicts and throughout the community.

Understanding the Reality of the Prescription Drug Misuse Problem

The stories of celebrities, ordinary American citizens, and entire communities destroyed by prescription drug misuse are both captivating and terrifying. The message conveyed is that everybody is at risk for prescription drug misuse, that prescription drug misuse is a significant threat to the social fabric of America, and that prescription drug misuse is an unstoppable force that is poised to tear apart all American communities. But do these seemingly isolated and sensationalized stories represent the reality of prescription drug misuse in the United States? Who is most likely to misuse prescription medications and why? Are trends in prescription drug use similar to or different from other forms of drug abuse? How do people begin misusing prescription drugs? What are the programs and policies that have been used to combat prescription drug misuse, and have those policies and programs been effective? What other steps can be taken to address this problem? Is there any hope for individuals and communities struggling with prescription drug misuse?

This book presents comprehensive answers to each of these questions. But to fully understand the prescription drug misuse problem and solutions, we must first understand the history of prescription drug misuse, the complexity in defining prescription drug misuse, the different categories of prescription drugs that are misused, and the types of data that are most often used by researchers to present an accurate picture of the scale and scope of the prescription drug misuse epidemic in the United States.

History of Prescription Drug Misuse

Although recent media and political attention on the current prescription drug misuse problem in the United States makes it appear that prescription drug misuse is new, the fact is that prescription drug misuse has been part of the American culture since at least the American Civil War. For example, morphine, a pain reliever derived from opium, was widely used to treat injury-related pain during the Civil War. So many soldiers became addicted to morphine that it became known as "Soldiers' Disease" following the war.[56] Partly due to the rampant abuse of morphine in the post–Civil War United States, the Harrison Act was passed in 1914, which mandated that any person involved with the distribution or manufacture of opium or coca leaves and related substances must be licensed by the U.S. government. The law also stipulated that physicians keep records of the drugs prescribed and dispensed. Morphine continues to be used to treat severe pain, mostly in hospitals through intravenous drip, but morphine can also be administered in a pill form that continues to be widely misused.

Similarly, amphetamines were originally used in the treatment of obesity, fatigue, and depression before being regulated by the U.S. government.

During World War II, soldiers would often use amphetamines to treat fatigue, which continues to be a main reason for amphetamine abuse in the United States today. College students, for example, will misuse amphetamines to study for exams or stay awake for late-night parties. Ritalin, a current form of amphetamine this is widely misused, was originally developed in 1954 to treat depression, fatigue, and narcolepsy. Ritalin (and the related drug Adderall) was developed to treat hyperactivity in children in the 1960s and continues to be prescribed to treat attention-deficit/hyperactivity disorder (ADHD). Ritalin and Adderall misuse is increasingly prevalent among high school and college students to stay awake and focused while studying, but these substances are also misused to get high and control weight.

Antianxiety medications are also ripe for misuse. In 1955, Miltown was released as a safer alternative for treating anxiety than prior medications that caused extreme drowsiness or included dangerous and deadly narcotics. In 1963, Valium was marketed to patients to treat anxiety and a variety of other conditions (i.e., alcohol withdrawal, convulsive disorders). Because Valium was used to treat such a wide variety of ailments, it has been one of the most widely prescribed and misused medications in the United States. At the peak of Valium popularity in 1978, 20 percent of all American women and 14 percent of all American men were taking the tranquilizer, making it the best-selling pharmaceutical medication in American history. The ubiquitous availability of the drug also made Valium one of the most frequently misused medications in U.S. history.

Among the major antecedents to the current American prescription drug misuse crisis was the development of fentanyl, a powerful opioid, in the 1960s. Fentanyl was originally administered intravenously, but many different forms of fentanyl have been marketed over the decades since it was released. The most common current form of fentanyl is a slow-release patch that is often stolen from hospitals and pharmacies; the patches are cut open to extract the fentanyl. More recently, drug manufacturers have developed lollipops and lozenges with fentanyl to work as a fast-acting pain reliever for cancer patients experiencing extreme pain. Fentanyl misuse was first noticed among medical professionals in the 1970s, and the lollipop version of fentanyl has been found in the illegal drug market with the nicknames "perc-a-pop" and "narco-pop."

In an attempt to treat pain without the severe addictive qualities of fentanyl, Talwin was released in 1967, but like so many pain-relieving medications released before, Talwin quickly became a staple of the illicit drug market. Because of its addictive qualities, Talwin was added to the

Controlled Substances Act as a Schedule IV drug in 1979 (accepted medical use and lower abuse potential than other medications with higher schedule ratings, such as Valium and Xanax). To counteract the addictive qualities and abuse potential of Talwin, Talwin Nix was created, which contained a substance, naloxone, that reduced the morphine-like effects of Talwin if the tablets were dissolved and injected. As a result, misuse of Talwin nearly stopped.[57]

Vicodin is another opioid pain reliever that has become widely misused. The primary ingredient in Vicodin is hydrocodone, which was originally developed in the 1920s as an alternative to other pain relievers that would be less toxic and harsh on the stomach. Like other opioids, Vicodin causes a powerful euphoria and is highly addictive, but unlike other opioids, tolerance to Vicodin develops more slowly, and withdrawal symptoms are not as severe. As Vicodin prescriptions have expanded since the early 1990s, Vicodin misuse and dependence have increased substantially.

All of the medications described above set the stage for potential prescription drug misuse, but the release of OxyContin in 1996 by Purdue Pharma is closely linked to the current prescription drug misuse crisis in the United States. OxyContin is a highly potent opioid that releases oxycodone over a 12-hour period, thus providing extended pain relief with fewer pills. Largely driven by an intense marketing campaign by Purdue Pharma, by 2001 OxyContin was the most frequently prescribed narcotic medication for moderate to severe pain in the United States. OxyContin prescriptions written to treat noncancer pain increased from 670,000 in 1997 to 6.2 million in 2002.[58] OxyContin diversion and misuse became rampant, especially in the Appalachia regions of Kentucky, Virginia, and West Virginia, but quickly spread across the entire United States.

Originally, the Food and Drug Administration allowed OxyContin to be sold with a label claiming that the drug had a lower addiction potential than other opioids because of the time-release formula. The label also included a safety warning not to crush the pills, because doing so would bypass the time-release mechanisms and expose the user to toxic levels of the drug. Ironically, this warning actually served as an instruction to drug misusers as to how to achieve the most potent high from OxyContin. OxyContin misusers routinely crush the pills and either snort or inject the medication for an immediate narcotic rush. One of the reasons for the rapid spread of OxyContin misuse is that the drug sells for up to 10 times its retail value on the black market, making it incredibly profitable for illicit drug sellers.[59]

Categories of Misused Prescription Medications

Definitions of prescription drug misuse vary, but the general way that surveys define prescription drug misuse as "use of prescription drugs that were not prescribed for an individual or were taken only for the experience of feeling that the drugs caused."[60] More recent updates have recognized that the general definition of prescription drug misuse, originally termed "nonmedical prescription drug use," does not include situations where prescription drugs prescribed to somebody else were misused to treat legitimate pain issues or the overuse of medications prescribed to an individual. In other words, the standard definition of prescription drug misuse provided conservative estimates of the problem. To remedy these concerns, descriptions of prescription drug misuse have shifted from "nonmedical use" to "prescription drug misuse" with a broader definition that includes "(1) use without a prescription of the respondent's own; (2) use in greater amounts, more often, or longer than the respondent was told to take them; or (3) use in any other way a doctor did not direct the respondent to use them."[61]

Any prescription medication can be misused, but the most commonly misused prescription drugs fall into one of four categories: pain relievers, tranquilizers, stimulants, and sedatives.

Pain Relievers

Although nonopioid pain relievers, such as anti-inflammatory prescription drugs, can be misused, relatively few people misuse them. Rather, nearly all misuse of prescription pain relievers includes opioid-based medications. Prescription opioids, also known as narcotics and analgesics, are prescribed to relieve pain, which is the most common complaint given to physicians.[62] Opioids are prescribed to treat acute pain, cancer-related chronic pain, and noncancer chronic pain and are therefore an important aspect of pain management. Opioids work by attaching to opioid receptors in the brain, effectively blocking pain signals to the brain. Opioids also produce an enhanced feeling of pleasure.

Opioid medications come in many different forms: hydrocodone (i.e., Lortab, Vicodin), oxycodone (i.e., OxyContin, Percocet), tramadol (i.e., Ultram), morphine (i.e., Avinza, Kadian), fentanyl (i.e., Actiq, Duragesic), buprenorphine (i.e., Suboxone), oxymorphone (i.e., Opana), Demerol, and hydromorphone (i.e., Dilaudid). Nearly all opioid-based pain relievers are classified as Schedule II drugs by the Controlled Substances Act, meaning that these drugs are considered to have legitimate medical uses with the highest abuse potential of any such drug. The exceptions are tramadol products, which are Schedule IV drugs (accepted medical use, lower abuse potential than most other prescription drugs), and buprenorphine products, which are Schedule III medications (accepted medical use with lower abuse potential than Schedule II drugs).

There is no doubt that prescription opioids are addictive, as with heroin (an opioid with no legitimate medical uses), but pain management specialists and addiction specialists often debate the degree to which prescribing opioid medications to treat acute chronic pain is a risk factor for opioid addiction. Because evidence of addiction resulting from legitimate prescribing practices is mixed, "physicians must walk the delicate line of balancing appropriate pain management while avoiding over-prescribing and patient addiction."[63]

The most significant consequence of long-term prescription opioid misuse is physical dependence on the drugs, which is characterized by increased tolerance to the drug and withdrawal symptoms when the drug use is reduced or stopped. People withdrawing from prescription opioid use often experience trouble sleeping, pain in bones and muscles, and severe diarrhea or vomiting. These withdrawal symptoms even occur when opioids are taken appropriately for medical purposes. When opioids are taken in large doses at one time, they can significantly slow breathing and lead to death.

Tranquilizers

Prescription tranquilizers are central nervous system (CNS) depressants used primarily to treat anxiety disorders or reduce muscle spasms. Tranquilizers influence the neurotransmitter gamma-aminobutyric acid to reduce or slow brain activity, therefore creating a calming effect. Prescription tranquilizers come in many forms, primarily benzodiazepines and muscle relaxants. Benzodiazepines include alprazolam (i.e., Xanax), lorazepam (i.e., Ativan), clonazepam (i.e., Klonopin), and diazepam (i.e., Valium). Muscle relaxants include cyclobenzaprine (i.e., Flexeril) and Soma. All tranquilizers are Schedule IV drugs in the Controlled Substances Act, meaning that they all have legitimate medical uses and have lower abuse potential than most other prescription medications. That said, certain benzodiazepines that are very potent and act quickly (i.e., Xanax) are more likely to lead to addiction than slower-acting benzodiazepines.[64] Long-term use of tranquilizers can lead to physical dependence whereby tolerance to the drug is increased and withdrawal symptoms occur when tranquilizer use is abruptly stopped. Withdrawal from tranquilizers often creates an intense need for more of the drug to produce the calming effect and can cause seizures. Death from tranquilizers is extremely rare except when they are used in combination with alcohol or other drugs.

Stimulants

Prescription stimulants enhance brain activity by increasing the neurotransmitters norepinephrine and dopamine. Stimulants increase alertness, concentration, and energy and cause increases in blood pressure and respiration rates. Additionally, prescription stimulants create euphoric sensations similar to illicit stimulants such as cocaine. Stimulants were originally developed to treat asthma and other respiratory problems as well as obesity, but physicians are increasingly choosing other medications to treat these disorders because of concerns about the abuse potential of prescription stimulants. Currently, prescription stimulants are primarily used to treat ADHD and narcolepsy. Prescription stimulants include amphetamines (i.e., Adderall), methylphenidate (i.e., Ritalin), anorectic stimulants used for weight loss (i.e., Didrex), and Provigil used to treat narcolepsy and other sleep disorders. The amphetamine (i.e., Adderall) and methylphenidate (i.e., Ritalin) products are Schedule II drugs in the Controlled Substances Act, meaning that the drugs have legitimate medical uses and have a high potential for abuse. The anorectic stimulants are Schedule III or IV drugs with legitimate medical uses and lower abuse potential, and Provigil is a Schedule IV substance with a lower abuse potential than most other drugs. Although there has been some debate as to whether long-term therapeutic use of Adderall and Ritalin leads to addiction or abuse, the general consensus is that the medical use of stimulants does not significantly increase the likelihood of later abuse.[65] Rather, most people who misuse prescription stimulants do not obtain the medications through legitimate sources.[66]

Physical dependence, including increased tolerance and withdrawal symptoms, can result from abuse of stimulant medications. Side effects of stimulant misuse range from dizziness to insomnia, rapid or irregular heartbeat, and high blood pressure. In extreme cases, stimulant misuse can cause paranoia, hallucinations, heart failure, or deadly seizures. Because of these side effects, prescription stimulant misusers will often attempt to counteract the effects of stimulants with CNS depressants (i.e., alcohol, benzodiazepines) or even opioids. Therefore, prescription stimulant misusers are also at a high risk of developing addictions to multiple substances.

Sedatives

Like prescription tranquilizers, prescription sedatives are also CNS depressants. Prescription sedatives are primarily used to treat sleep disorders such as insomnia by decreasing brain activity and reducing the activity of muscle tissues, including the heart and the respiratory system. Sedatives are prescribed to induce anesthesia or sleep. Prescription sedatives include zolpidem (i.e., Ambien), eszopiclone (i.e., Lunesta), and zaleplon (i.e., Sonata). There are also benzodiazepine sedatives, including flurazepam, tamazepam (i.e., Restoril), and triazolam (i.e., Halcion). Finally, barbiturate sedatives include Butisol, Seconal, and phenobarbital. Medical use of benzodiazepine sedatives has become much more popular in recent years than barbiturate sedatives, as the benzodiazepine sedatives are more effective and have a much lower risk of coma or death than barbiturates. Abrupt cessation of prescription sedatives increases the risk of severe withdrawal symptoms, including hallucinations and even death, especially with barbiturates. As with the benzodiazepine tranquilizers described above, death from prescription benzodiazepine sedative abuse is very unlikely except when the sedatives are taken with alcohol or other drugs.

Most prescription sedatives have a low risk of abuse, classified as Schedule IV drugs in the Controlled Substances Act. The exception is that some barbiturates are classified as Schedule II (Seconal) with a high abuse potential or Schedule III (Butisol) with lower abuse potential than Seconal and higher abuse potential than other barbiturates such as phenobarbital, which is a Schedule IV drug.

Types of Data Used to Study Prescription Drug Abuse

Depending on the population addressed in research on prescription drug abuse, there are numerous nationwide data sources to analyze. For instance, Monitoring the Future is a nationally representative sample of 8th, 10th, and 12th graders in the United States collected each year since 1975. The survey began by sampling only 12th graders (1975–1990), with 8th and 10th graders added to the survey in 1991. Monitoring the Future surveys approximately 50,000 high school students each year. The survey includes detailed questions about alcohol, tobacco, and drug use and is widely used in to track trends in youth substance use over time. Another survey, the Harvard School of Public Health College Alcohol Study, focuses mainly on substance use patterns among college students. The study was conducted in 1993, 1997, 1999, and 2001 and includes over

14,000 students at 120 colleges in 40 U.S. states. This study was among the first to highlight the problems of binge drinking on college campuses but has also been used to establish correlates of prescription drug misuse among college students.[67]

Although we will occasionally refer to both Monitoring the Future and the Harvard School of Public Health College Alcohol Survey throughout this book, the main source of data we will use to highlight trends in prescription drug misuse over time is the National Survey on Drug Use and Health (NSDUH). Collected every year since 1971, NSDUH is the most comprehensive, nationwide survey of drug use currently available. NSDUH is a survey of the U.S. population ages 12 and above, excluding Americans in the military or in an institution such as a prison or hospital. This means that the results of the survey are representative of the entire civilian, noninstitutionalized U.S. population ages 12 and older.

Although the NSDUH data are perfectly suited for establishing long-term trends in drug abuse, there were some important changes to the survey over the years that limit comparability of drug use estimates from different time periods. In 1994, for instance, a new questionnaire was used, and new data editing and imputation techniques were introduced. Therefore, information before and after 1994 must be interpreted cautiously. The data used for this book begins with the 1994 survey. In 1999, the survey switched from paper-and-pencil form to computer-assisted form. Because people tend to be more open and honest about their behaviors on computer-assisted surveys, especially drug use, comparisons between 1999 and later surveys with earlier surveys need to be interpreted with caution.

In 2002, additional significant changes were made to the survey. First, the name of the survey was changed from the National Household Survey on Drug Abuse, as it was called from 1971 to 2001, to the NSDUH. Second, a $30 incentive was offered to respondents starting with the 2002 survey, which greatly increased response rates. Third, better training and quality-control practices were implemented in the 2002 and later surveys. Finally, the population data used to weight the survey responses was based on the 2000 U.S. census information beginning in 2002. Taken together, these changes in the 2002 and later surveys limit the ability to compare population estimates of substance use and many other measures from the 2002 and later surveys to earlier surveys.

Because of the many changes to the survey over the past 20 years, the analyses presented in this book show trends separately for 1994–1998, 1999–2001, and 2002–2014. Because the survey changes appear to have influenced reporting patterns similarly for all demographic groups, however, we will occasionally refer to overall changes in drug use patterns from 1994 to 2014. These percentage changes cannot be interpreted independently, but the magnitude of the changes can be used to show that drug use patterns evolved differently for the various subgroups identified in the analyses.

CHAPTER ONE

The New American Drug Epidemic?

As we detailed in the prior chapter, there are countless stories of death and despair caused by prescription drug abuse among celebrities, ordinary Americans, and entire communities. These stories are sad and worrisome, but do these stories represent the reality of prescription drug misuse in the United States? After all, it is possible that these stories of prescription drug misuse are isolated to small groups of Americans or are overly sensationalized to attract readers or viewers to media sources—as was evident during the crack scare of the 1980s. It is also possible that the trends in prescription drug use simply mirror trends in the use of other illicit drugs. In this chapter, we present a comprehensive review of research on the trends and correlates of prescription drug misuse in the United States, primarily over the past two decades, to illustrate the scope and scale of the prescription drug misuse problem.

To answer some of these questions, we rely on two important sources of data. The first source of data that we draw upon is the National Survey on Drug Use and Health (NSDUH), which is a nationally representative sample of noninstitutionalized Americans ages 12 and older. This means that the prevalence rates and trends in prescription drug misuse as well as the abuse of other drugs can be generalized to the entire U.S. population ages 12 and older. At the time of this writing, the latest publicly available data from the NSDUH was collected in 2014. To show the long-term trends in drug use, we start with the 1994 version of the NSDUH and include drug use estimates from every yearly NSDUH through the 2014 data.

Prevalence rates over time, however, are only part of the prescription drug use story in the United States. As we illustrated in the stories of celebrities, ordinary Americans, and communities that have been afflicted with the prescription drug misuse scourge, drug overdose deaths are also part of the U.S. drug use problem. To show the long-term trends in drug overdose deaths, we also draw upon data from the Centers for Disease Control and Prevention (CDC) that is made publicly available through the Wonder database. CDC Wonder classifies the primary cause of death for every death that occurs in the United States on a yearly basis, including categories of drug overdose deaths. The publicly available data in CDC Wonder begins in 1999, and data are currently available through 2015.

We first present what the data show about the current state of the prescription drug misuse problem in the United States, including several measures of overall prevalence use rates and death rates as well as prevalence use rates and death rates among specific populations of Americans. Specifically, we document the drug use and death patterns by sex, race, age, and rural or urban residence. Income will be the focus of a later chapter. We then focus on the long-term patterns of prescription drug misuse and death for the United States overall and for the specific demographic groups to better show how we arrived at the current state of drug misuse in the United States. Throughout the descriptions of the current and long-term drug use patterns, comparisons are made to the same patterns of marijuana and hard drug use to determine if the prescription drug problems currently facing the United States are unique or developed along with the use of other types of drugs.

Ultimately, by focusing on the current state of the prescription drug misuse problem, the long-term trends in prescription drug misuse, and the prescription drug misuse patterns by demographic groups in the United States, the goal is to better identify the potential causes of—and possible solutions to—the prescription drug misuse problem.

The Current State of Prescription Drug Misuse in the United States

The NSDUH shows that nearly 27 million Americans ages 12 or older were considered current illicit drug users in 2014, defined as having used any illicit substance (including *misusing* any prescription medication) in the month prior to the survey. Stated more clearly, 1 out of every 10 Americans used at least one illicit drug in the past month. Of these 27 million people who reported having used a drug in the past month, 6.5 million were considered current prescription drug misusers, or 2.3 percent of the U.S. population. In comparison, just over 3 million Americans, or

1.2 percent of the U.S. population, were current users of cocaine, heroin, hallucinogens, and inhalants *combined*, known as "hard drugs." Further, more than 22 million Americans, or 8.3 percent of the U.S. population, were current marijuana users. Marijuana is therefore the most commonly used drug in the United States, but prescription drugs are the second most commonly abused category of drugs. To put the scale of the prescription drug misuse problem in perspective, there are more than double the number of prescription drug misusers in the United States than users of all hard drugs *combined*.

Among the four categories of prescription drugs that are most often misused (pain killers, tranquilizers, stimulants, and sedatives), the most striking prescription drug misuse problem by far is the misuse of prescription pain relievers. Of the 6.5 million past-month prescription drug misusers in 2014, 4.3 million, or 1.3 percent of the U.S. population, were current prescription pain medication misusers. Two-thirds of current prescription drug misusers in 2014 misused prescription pain relievers. Nearly all the prescription pain reliever misuse in 2014 involved opioid-based medications. In contrast, there were 1.8 million prescription tranquilizer misusers (0.7 percent of the U.S. population), 1.4 million prescription stimulant misusers (0.5 percent of the U.S. population), and 270,000 prescription sedative misusers (0.1 percent of the U.S. population) in 2014. Please note that the numbers do not add to the 6.5 million current prescription drug users reported above, as many people report abusing more than one category of prescription medications in any given year, an issue we explore in detail later in this chapter.

Past-month drug use statistics, however, only provide estimates of the percentage of the population that was *currently* using each type of drug at the time of the survey. The NSDUH also provides past-year and past-month prevalence use numbers for the U.S. population. Whereas 2.3 percent of the U.S. population misused a prescription medication in the past month in 2014, 6.3 percent reported past-year misuse of a prescription medication, and 20 percent reported ever having misused a prescription drug. This means that approximately 54 million Americans have misused a prescription medication at some point during their lives and that 17 million Americans reported past-year prescription drug misuse in 2014. In comparison, 3.3 percent of Americans reported having used a hard drug in the past year, and 22.1 percent reported having ever used a hard drug. For marijuana, 13.3 percent reported past-year marijuana use, and 44.2 percent reported having ever used marijuana. Although marijuana is by far the most commonly used drug in the United States, it is important to stress that in the 2014 survey more Americans reported having ever used a hard drug than reported having ever misused a prescription medication. Despite the higher lifetime prevalence rate for hard drugs rather than prescription drug misuse, roughly double the number of Americans reported past-year or past-month prescription drug misuse than hard drug use in 2014.

The ever, past-year, and past-month prevalence rates and patterns raise the possibility that the continuation of drug use varies by the type of drug used. To represent the continuation of drug use, we created a "stickiness" measure for calculating the percentage of Americans who reported having ever used each type of drug and also reported past-month use of that drug.

In 2014, of the 54 million Americans who reported having ever misused a prescription drug, 11.5 percent reported past-month prescription drug misuse. In short, 1 out of every 9 people who reported having misused a prescription painkiller, sedative, stimulant, or tranquilizer reported past-month prescription drug misuse in 2014.

Marijuana, however, shows a much higher rate of stickiness than prescription drug misuse. Of the 44.2 percent of the U.S. population (roughly 117 million people) ages 12 and older who reported having ever used marijuana, 18.9 percent report past-month marijuana use. Essentially, a little less than 1 out of every 5 Americans who have experimented with marijuana at least once reported past-month marijuana use in the 2014 NSDUH. Contrary to popular belief, hard drugs show a lower degree of stickiness than either marijuana or prescription drug misuse. Of the nearly 60 million Americans who have ever used cocaine, heroin, crack, inhalants, or hallucinogens, only 5.3 percent reported past-month hard drug use in the 2014 survey. Approximately 1 out of every 20 people in the United States who has experimented with hard drugs at some point in their life becomes a past-month or past-year hard drug user.

A Focus on Prescription Opioid Misuse

Opioid addiction dominates public attention on the current drug misuse crisis facing the United States. Indeed, prescription drug misuse in the United States is dominated by the misuse of prescription painkillers, the overwhelming majority of which involves opiate-based medications. Of the nearly 54 million people in the United States who have misused a prescription medication at some point during their lives, more that 34 million have ever misused a prescription opioid painkiller. This means that two-thirds of people who have ever misused a prescription medication misused an opiate-based painkiller. Importantly, among the 15 million Americans who reported past-year prescription drug misuse in 2014,

9 million people, or 60 percent, reported past-year prescription painkiller misuse. Focusing on the 6.3 million Americans who reported past-month prescription drug misuse in 2014, 4.3 million, or 67.7 percent, reported past-month prescription painkiller misuse. Stated simply, the prescription drug misuse problem in the United States is largely a prescription opioid misuse problem.

In contrast, hard drug use was not nearly as dominated by opioid use (i.e., heroin) as was evident with the prescription drug misuse problem in 2014. Among the 60 million Americans who have used a hard drug at least once in their lives, only 5 million, or 8.3 percent of ever hard drug users, reported having ever used heroin. Among the 9 million Americans who reported past-year hard drug use, 1 million, or 11.2 percent of past-year hard drug users, reported heroin use in 2014. Focusing specifically on the 3 million past-month hard drug users, 462,000 used heroin, which represents 15.4 percent of the past-month hard drug users. Opioids clearly dominate the current prescription drug misuse crisis in the United States, but heroin use is a more minor contributor to hard drug use in the United States. That said, the data do signify that heroin is more common among regular past-month hard drug users than among those who use hard drugs sporadically (i.e., in the past year) or experimentally (i.e., ever used).

The addictive properties of prescription opiates are well known, and similar to the "instantaneous addiction" claims during the crack cocaine scare, it is widely believed that prescription opiates are highly likely to be addictive to those who experiment with the drug. The 2014 data showed that 28 percent of people who had ever misused a prescription painkiller reported past-year prescription painkiller misuse, and 11.6 percent reported past-month prescription painkiller misuse. With heroin, 20.4 percent of those who had ever used heroin reported past-year heroin use in 2014, while 9.4 percent reported past-month heroin use. The vast majority of people who have misused an opioid, whether in prescription or heroin form, at some point in their past do not continue to misuse opioids, but prescription opioid misuse is slightly more "sticky" than heroin.

Although the data show that opioid misuse is not as sticky as public impression might suggest, the stickiness of prescription opiates and heroin must be put in context. As mentioned in the prior chapter, Reinarman and Levine reported that a 1992 national survey—a survey taken at the end of the crack scare—showed that only 3 percent of people between 18 and 35 years of age had ever used crack cocaine.[1] Further, Reinarman and Levine report that only about one-third of those who had ever used crack cocaine reported use of the drug in the prior year, and only about

10 percent had used crack in the past month. Therefore, in comparison to crack cocaine, prescription drugs generally and prescription opioids specifically are a much larger problem than crack cocaine ever was. It is also important to note that the data on crack use was focused only on 18–35-year-olds, the demographic most likely to use drugs, but the prescription drug misuse data includes the entire population of the United States ages 12 and older. Six to seven times more Americans have at least experimented with prescription drug misuse than occurred with crack cocaine during the height of the crack scare, and similarly higher proportions of the population continue to misuse prescription medications on a past-year or past-month basis, compared to similar measures of crack from the 1992 survey. Although crack and prescription opioid medication misuse is equally sticky, with 10–11 percent of "ever" users continuing regular misuse of both substances, the sheer magnitude of the prescription drug misuse problem is far greater than any measure of crack use during the 1980s scare.

Compared with other forms of drug use in the 2014 data, prescription opioid misuse was also a noteworthy problem. First, a greater proportion of Americans had misused a prescription opioid (13.6 percent) at some point in the past than any other drug except for marijuana (44.2 percent), cocaine (14.8 percent), and hallucinogens (15 percent). More strikingly, however, a greater percentage of the American population reported past-year and past-month prescription opioid misuse than any other drug besides marijuana. In fact, there were more past-year and past-month prescription opioid misusers in the United States than past-year or past-month users of hard drugs *combined*. Prescription opioid misuse was also "stickier" than all other drugs except for marijuana—a larger percentage of Americans who have experimented with prescription opiate misuse continue to misuse the medication on a past-month basis than any other illicit hard drug or class of prescription medication. The next closest drug in terms of stickiness is heroin, which of course is also an opiate drug with chemical properties that are similar to the prescription opioid medications. Although heroin will be a focus in subsequent chapters, it must be noted that even though heroin is a sticky drug in terms of habitual and/or regular use, far fewer Americans have experimented with heroin than prescription opiates. To illustrate, while 34 million Americans have ever misused a prescription opioid medication, fewer than 5 million Americans have ever used heroin.

That data shows that prescription opiate misuse is a major problem in the United States, affecting millions more Americans than crack ever did even during the height of the crack frenzy in the 1980s, and that millions more Americans misuse prescription opioids than all other hard drugs combined. Further, prescription opioids are much stickier than crack during the crack scare and than any other hard drug or prescription medication misused in the most recent data. That said, prescription opiates are misused by only 1.6 percent of the American population on a past-month basis, quite far from reaching proportions that meet any standard definition of an epidemic. The roots of the public concern, media coverage, and political attention to the prescription drug misuse problem in the United States, however, might not be based on the sheer numbers of users; rather, the reason for concern very well might be the severe consequences of prescription drug misuse—namely overdose deaths—that will be discussed in detail later in this chapter.

The question remains, however, have prescription drug misuse prevalence rates increased over the past two decades? If so, have prescription drug misuse prevalence rates increased faster than the use of other drugs? The trends in prescription drug misuse will help determine if the United States has developed a specific prescription drug misuse problem or a more general problem with all forms of drug use. Overall, the trends described below serve as evidence to inform whether the United States is actually experiencing a prescription drug misuse epidemic.

The Precipitous Prescription Drug Misuse Explosion?

Due to the changes in data-collection methodologies in the NSDUH over the past 20 years described in the previous chapter, the trends in drug use from 1994 to 2014 are broken into specific time periods: 1994–1998, 1999–2001, and 2002–2014. Comparisons cannot be made between the specific time periods, but each of the tables describing changes in drug misuse do include an overall percentage change in drug use from 1994 to 2014. Assuming that the data-collection changes by the NSDUH in 1999 and 2002 influenced the reporting patterns for all groups of Americans and for each form of drug use equally, the overall percentage change in drug misuse from 1994 to 2014 is useful only for comparison purposes. Although the overall percentage changes in drug misuse cannot be interpreted, the relative magnitude of changes can be examined to identify the groups that experienced more or less of an increase in drug use across this period.

In 1994, only 0.5 percent of the U.S. population reported having misused a prescription medication in the past month. By 2014, the percentage of the U.S. population who reported past-month prescription drug misuse reached 2.3 percent. Even with the methodological changes in the data collection that increased reporting rates, it cannot be denied that the United States witnessed a profound increase in percentage of the population who reported past-month prescription drug misuse over the past 20 years. The increase in the past-month prevalence rate of prescription drug misuse, however, was not steady across this 20-year period. From 1994 to 1998, the percentage of the population who reported past-month prescription drug misuse increased 55 percent. The period from 1999 to 2001 also showed an increase in prescription drug misuse of 21 percent. From 2002 to 2014, however, the prevalence of past-month prescription drug misuse deceased by 10 percent. Prescription drug misuse therefore increased rapidly in the late 1990s and throughout the 2000s to a peak of 2.7 percent in 2009, but prescription drug misuse rates have noticeably decreased in recent years.

Past-month marijuana use and hard drug use prevalence rates also increased rapidly between 1994 and 2014, but the rate of increase was not as rapid for marijuana and hard drugs as was seen for prescription drug misuse. In 1994, 2.4 percent of the U.S. population reported past-month marijuana use, which increased to 7.4 percent of the U.S. population in 2014. Again, even accounting for the methodological changes by the NSDUH, it is obvious that past-month marijuana use prevalence rates increased dramatically across this 20-year period. Compared with prescription drug misuse prevalence rate increases, however, past-month marijuana use prevalence rates increased at a slower pace. Additionally, it is important to note that the increases in marijuana use show a different pattern than increases in prescription drug misuse. From 1994 to 1998 past-month marijuana use rates increased by 37.9 percent, which is a slower rate of increase than prescription drug misuse during the same period. From 1999 to 2001 past-month marijuana use rates increased by 14.2 percent, which is also slower than the increases in past-month prescription drug misuse rates during that period. Notably, past-month marijuana use rates increased rapidly from 2002 to 2014, a period when past-month prescription drug misuse rates decreased. The rise in marijuana use over the past 20 years was therefore slower than the rise in past-month prescription drug misuse rates, but marijuana use continued to increase in recent years even when past-month prescription drug misuse was declining.

The percentage of the U.S. population who reported past-month hard drug use also increased over the past 20 years, but the increase in hard drug use was much slower than the increases in prescription drug misuse and marijuana use. In 1994 past-month hard drug use was slightly more common in the United States than prescription drug misuse, but by 2014 past-month hard drug use was about half as common as past-month prescription drug misuse. Although past-month hard drug use in the United States did increase over the past 20 years, past-month prescription drug misuse increased much more rapidly than hard drug use. Similar to prescription drug misuse patterns in the United States and in contrast to marijuana use patterns, past-month hard drug use in the United States decreased noticeably between 2002 and 2014.

The data clearly shows that the overall drug use prevalence rates have increased substantially over the past 20 years, but prescription drug misuse prevalence rates increased much more rapidly than either marijuana or hard drug use. It is also worth noting that the three categories of drug use follow much different patterns. Prescription drug misuse did not follow patterns similar to either hard drug use or marijuana use over the past 20 years. Rather, it appears that prescription drug misuse emerged as an independent category of drug use that is not influenced by the same forces that drive marijuana or hard drug use. Prescription drug misuse emerged as a unique category of drug misuse during a period of across-the-board increases in drug use in the United States.

Because prescription opioid medications dominate the prescription drug misuse problem, the increase in past-month prescription drug misuse over the past 20 years was, not surprisingly, largely attributed to rapid increases in prescription opioid misuse. In 1994, 0.3 percent of the U.S. population reported past-month prescription painkiller misuse, which amounted to 60 percent of all prescription drug misuse in that year. Between 1994 and 1998 past-month prescription opioid misuse nearly doubled, and prescription opioid medication misuse accounted for a greater percentage of all prescription drug misuse in 1998. Between 1999 and 2001, past-month prescription opioid misuse continued to increase. From 2002 to 2014, prescription opioid misuse decreased by 14 percent, and prescription opioids accounted for a lower percentage of past-month prescription drug misuse. The rise and fall of past-month prescription drug misuse prevalence rates therefore depends largely on the rise and fall of past-month prescription opioid misuse.

Although the prevalence rate for past-month heroin use was much lower than the prevalence rate for prescription opioid misuse, the chemical similarities between the two types of drugs demand a similar evaluation of trends for heroin use over the past 20 years. In 1994, only 0.1 percent of the U.S. population reported past-month heroin use. By 1998, the past-month prevalence rate for heroin use dropped by half. Further reductions in past-month heroin use occurred between 1999 and 2001. The period between 2002 and 2014, however, showed a rapid resurgence in heroin use, with past-month heroin use more than doubling during that period. That said, only 0.2 percent of the U.S. population reported past-month heroin use in 2014.

Clearly, prescription drug misuse increased substantially over the past 20 years. To be sure, the use of marijuana and other hard drugs increased dramatically during this period as well, but the rate of increase for prescription drug misuse far outpaced growth in the use of other drugs. As a proportion of the U.S. population, there were almost five times the number of past-month prescription drug misusers in 2014 than there were in 1994, whereas there were more than three times the number of marijuana users and about twice the number of hard drug users. Some of the increases in prescription drug misusers during this period are due to the methodological changes by the NSDUH during the past 20 years, but it is clear that prescription drug misuse has grown rapidly during this period. To be sure, drug use increased across the board, but prescription drug misuse obviously grew at a much more rapid pace than any of the other drugs. In contrast to the crack scare, where no empirical evidence showed rapid increases in cocaine or crack use, the public concern about the current prescription drug misuse problem is warranted and supported by the data.

To better understand the prescription drug misuse crisis, a full investigation of the demographic trends in prescription drug misuse is needed. The goal of the following analyses is to determine if the prescription drug misuse problem is widespread, affecting everybody equally, or is concentrated among specific groups of people in the United States. By knowing which groups have been more or less affected by the prescription drug misuse crisis, we can better understand the social factors that have contributed to the prescription drug misuse problem in the United States and the public reactions to the prescription drug misuse crisis. Importantly, with a better understanding of the demographic distribution of prescription drug misuse problems and the possible social factors that have contributed, better treatment and prevention strategies can be identified and implemented.

Who Are the Prescription Drug Misusers?

Past drug use epidemics have largely been driven by males, poor people, racial/ethnic minorities, and urban areas. Does the prescription drug misuse crisis follow these same demographic trends? Determining the demographic correlates and trends of prescription drug misuse, compared with other forms of drug use, will help us better understand how and why the public and political response to the prescription drug misuse crisis has been different from prior drug scares. In this section, we use the 2014 national data to show how the current and past demographics of prescription drug misuse compared to other drug use patterns.

Gender

Table 1 provides a breakdown of the 2014 ever, past-year, and past-month drug use patterns as well as the stickiness measure that reflects the percentage of people by sex, income, race, age, education, and urban/rural location who have tried the drug at least once in their life and continue to use it on a regular basis. In general, males are more likely than females to use drugs in all forms. Compared with marijuana and hard drugs, however, males and females were nearly equally likely to have misused prescription medications in 2014. Although males are generally more likely than females to use drugs, the gender gap in prescription drug misuse is minuscule. In contrast to the past-month prescription drug misuse prevalence estimates that show virtually no difference between males and females, males were roughly 80 percent more likely than females to be current marijuana users and twice as likely to be current hard drug users in 2014.

Focusing specifically on prescription painkiller misuse, the same gendered pattern exists as with the overall prescription drug misuse problem. In 2014 the gender gap in prescription painkiller misuse was very narrow, especially in comparison to other forms of drug misuse. In contrast, males were twice as likely as females to have reported using heroin during the past month. Prescription painkiller misuse therefore shows a very narrow gender gap, but the gender gap in heroin use was much larger and closer to the gender gap in the use of marijuana and other hard drugs. It certainly appears that the demographics of the current prescription drug misuse crisis are different from other forms of drug use and different from past drug use crises, at least in terms of the gendered nature of the problem.

Another noteworthy aspect of the gendered nature of prescription drug misuse is the gender gap in the stickiness of prescription drug misuse compared to marijuana and hard drugs. The 2014 data show that a slightly higher percentage of females than males who have ever misused a prescription medication reported past-month prescription drug misuse. Not only was the gender gap in prescription drug misuse basically zero, but the data also show that females were *more* likely than males to continue prescription drug misuse. In contrast, both marijuana and hard drugs were slightly more sticky for males than females. Focusing

Table 1 Past-Month Prevalence of Drug Use, 2014

	2014 Marijuana Use				2014 Hard Drug Use				2014 Prescription Drug Misuse			
	Ever Used	Past Year Use	Past Month Use	Past Month Use/Ever Used	Ever Used	Past Year Use	Past Month Use	Past Month Use/Ever Used	Ever Used	Past Year Use	Past Month Use	Past Month Use/Ever Used
Sex												
Male	49.5%	16.5%	10.8%	21.9%	27.3%	4.4%	1.6%	5.7%	22.1%	5.8%	2.4%	11.0%
Female	39.3%	10.3%	6.0%	15.3%	17.2%	2.3%	0.8%	4.6%	18.3%	5.1%	2.2%	12.2%
Race												
White	49.3%	13.8%	8.7%	17.7%	25.5%	3.4%	1.1%	4.4%	23.1%	5.6%	2.3%	10.1%
Black	42.4%	15.9%	10.4%	24.5%	14.8%	2.9%	1.1%	7.5%	14.6%	5.2%	2.6%	17.9%
Hispanic	32.2%	11.0%	6.5%	20.1%	17.3%	3.4%	1.4%	8.1%	15.2%	5.5%	2.3%	14.9%
Age												
12–17	16.4%	12.8%	7.1%	43.1%	7.2%	3.4%	1.0%	14.4%	9.2%	5.7%	2.4%	26.0%
18–25	53.2%	31.9%	19.5%	36.7%	22.0%	9.2%	2.8%	12.7%	26.1%	11.3%	4.0%	15.2%
26–34	55.6%	20.2%	12.5%	22.4%	28.5%	5.8%	2.2%	7.6%	28.6%	8.7%	4.0%	13.9%
35–49	50.1%	11.1%	7.5%	15.0%	27.7%	2.5%	1.1%	4.0%	22.1%	5.1%	2.3%	10.4%
50+	40.4%	6.1%	4.0%	9.9%	20.2%	0.9%	0.4%	1.7%	16.5%	2.5%	1.2%	7.2%
Education												
Less than high school	36.5%	13.0%	8.6%	23.6%	20.1%	3.0%	1.0%	5.1%	19.3%	6.9%	3.1%	16.3%
High school	45.9%	13.7%	9.6%	20.9%	22.7%	3.1%	1.1%	4.7%	20.0%	4.9%	2.2%	10.8%
Some college	52.1%	16.1%	10.2%	19.6%	27.2%	4.2%	1.6%	5.9%	24.2%	6.4%	2.9%	12.0%
College grad	48.4%	10.7%	5.8%	12.1%	22.9%	1.0%	1.0%	4.2%	20.6%	4.4%	1.6%	7.7%

Population												
1 Million +	44.5%	13.8%	8.6%	19.2%	22.7%	3.6%	1.4%	6.0%	20.4%	5.6%	2.5%	12.0%
Less than 1 million	44.9%	13.1%	8.3%	18.4%	22.2%	3.1%	1.0%	4.5%	20.5%	5.5%	2.3%	11.0%
Not SMA or CMSA	36.8%	9.9%	6.7%	18.2%	16.0%	1.5%	0.5%	3.4%	15.0%	3.5%	1.7%	11.2%
Total	44.2%	13.3%	8.3%	18.9%	22.1%	3.3%	1.2%	5.3%	20.1%	6.3%	2.3%	11.5%

Source: 2014 NSDUH.

specifically on opioids, prescription painkillers were slightly more sticky for females than males in the 2014 data, and heroin was much stickier for females than males. In general, the data suggest that the gender gap in prescription drug misuse was much smaller than the gender gap in marijuana and hard drug use and that females are actually more likely to continue prescription opioid misuse and heroin use than males. Prescription drug misuse generally and opioid use or misuse specifically have affected females to a greater degree than other forms of drug use.

Trends in prescription drug abuse from 1994 to 2014 by gender and other demographic groups are shown in Table 2. In 1994 females were more likely to report past-month prescription drug misuse than males, but over the subsequent 20 years the gendered pattern of prescription drug misuse switched. The increase in prescription drug misuse from 1994 to 1998 was much more substantial for males than females. By 1998, males were about 50 percent more likely than females to report past-month prescription drug misuse, and although the gender gap in prescription drug misuse narrowed after 1998, with males being slightly more likely to misuse prescription medications than females, males remained more likely to report past-month prescription drug misuse in all years after 1998. Between 1999 and 2001 the increase in prescription drug misuse was more rapid among females than males, but from 2002 to 2014 the decrease in past-month prescription drug misuse prevalence rates was twice as fast among females than males. In general, past-month prescription drug misuse prevalence rates increased much more rapidly among males than females over the 20-year period between 1994 and 2014.

As shown in Tables 3 and 4, in contrast to the patterns of prescription drug misuse over the past 20 years, males have consistently been around 80 percent more likely to report past-month marijuana use and approximately twice as likely to report past-month hard drug use than females over this period. The gendered trends in marijuana and hard drug use also followed similar patterns across the three periods in this study. Between 1994 and 2014, both marijuana and hard drug use prevalence rates increased more rapidly for males than females, and between 1999 and 2001, the prevalence rate for both forms of drug use increased more substantially for females than males. Importantly, however, as marijuana use prevalence rates increased more rapidly for females than males between 2002 and 2014, hard drug use prevalence rates during this period decreased more rapidly for males than females. Despite the more rapid adoption of marijuana and hard drug use among females than males from 1994 to 2001 and the less rapid decrease in hard drug use among females from 2002 to 2014, males continued to be twice as likely

Table 2. Past-Month Prescription Drug Misuse, 1994–2014

	% Change 1994–1998	% Change 1999–2001	% Change 2002–2014	% Change 1994–2014
Sex				
Male	130.0%	15.7%	–6.9%	507.5%
	(0.40%–0.92%)	(1.78%–2.06%)	(2.61%–2.43%)	(0.40%–2.43%)
Female	6.9%	25.0%	–12.9%	282.8%
	(0.58%–0.62%)	(1.52%–1.90%)	(2.55%–2.22%)	(0.58%–2.22%)
Race				
White	57.4%	25.7%	–15.2%	333.3%
	(0.54%–0.85%)	(1.71%–2.15%)	(2.76%–2.34%)	(0.54%–2.34%)
Black	44.4%	6.1%	38.6%	627.8%
	(0.36%–0.52%)	(1.31%–1.39%)	(1.89%–2.62%)	(0.36%–2.62%)
Hispanic	31.1%	–3.6%	–17.8%	402.2%
	(0.45%–0.59%)	(1.65%–1.59%)	(2.75%–2.26%)	(0.45%–2.26%)
Age				
12–17	18.3%	16.8%	–32.5%	119.3%
	(1.09%–1.29%)	(2.44%–2.85%)	(3.54%–2.39%)	(1.09%–2.39%)
18–25	58.7%	32.7%	–25.7%	215.1%
	(1.26%–2.00%)	(3.49%–4.63%)	(5.34%–3.97%)	(1.26%–3.97%)
26–34	7.8%	65.7%	12.1%	343.3%
	(0.90%–0.97%)	(1.37%–2.27%)	(3.56%–3.99%)	(0.90%–3.99%)
35–49	476.9%	10.9%	–7.3%	1669.2%
	(0.13%–0.75%)	(1.83%–2.03%)	(2.48%–2.30%)	(0.13%–2.30%)
50+	–60.0%	–16.1%	41.7%	2280.0%
	(0.05%–0.02%)	(0.62%–0.52%)	(0.84%–1.19%)	(0.05%–1.19%)

(continued)

Table 2. *(continued)*

	% Change 1994–1998	% Change 1999–2001	% Change 2002–2014	% Change 1994–2014
Education				
Less than high school	–6.7%	37.0%	6.1%	199.0%
	(1.05%–0.98%)	(1.81%–2.48%)	(2.96%–3.14%)	(1.05%–3.14%)
High school	46.5%	50.4%	–17.6%	400.0%
	(0.43%–0.63%)	(1.39%–2.09%)	(2.61%–2.15%)	(0.43%–2.15%)
Some college	232.1%	22.4%	0.7%	942.9%
	(0.28%–0.93%)	(1.65%–2.02%)	(2.90%–2.92%)	(0.28%–2.92%)
College graduate	375.0%	–27.5%	4.6%	1875.0%
	(0.08%–0.38%)	(1.49%–1.08%)	(1.51%–1.58%)	(0.08%–1.58%)
Population				
1 million +	40.5%	12.8%	21.3%	483.3%
	(0.42%–0.59%)	(1.79%–2.02%)	(2.02%–2.45%)	(0.42%–2.45%)
Less than 1 million	128.9%	22.0%	–22.9%	400.0%
	(0.45%–1.03%)	(1.64%–2.00%)	(2.92%–2.25%)	(0.45%–2.25%)
Not SMA or CMSA	–2.9%	41.0%	–26.6%	140.0%
	(0.70%–0.68%)	(1.34%–1.89%)	(2.29%–1.68%)	(0.70%–1.68%)
Total	55.1%	20.7%	–10.1%	373.5%
	(0.49%–0.76%)	(1.64%–1.98%)	(2.58%–2.32%)	(0.49%–2.32%)

Source: 1994–2014 NSDUH.

Table 3. Past-Month Marijuana Use, 1994–2014

	% Change 1994–1998	% Change 1999–2001	% Change 2002–2014	% Change 1994–2014
Sex				
Male	74.0%	8.9%	36.4%	260.7%
	(3.00%–5.22%)	(6.26%–6.82%)	(7.93%–10.82%)	(3.00%–10.82%)
Female	63.4%	25.0%	41.0%	244.0%
	(1.75%–2.86%)	(3.00%–3.75%)	(4.27%–6.02%)	(1.75%–6.02%)
Race				
White	93.4%	21.1%	36.3%	91.0%
	(2.11%–4.08%)	(4.55%–5.51%)	(6.41%–8.74%)	(2.11%–8.74%)
Black	35.5%	–4.2%	47.1%	198.0%
	(3.49%–4.73%)	(5.52%–5.29%)	(7.07%–10.40%)	(3.49%–10.40%)
Hispanic	62.8%	–1.0%	55.8%	225.6%
	(1.99%–3.24%)	(4.02%–3.98%)	(4.16%–6.48%)	(1.99%–6.48%)
Age				
12–17	136.7%	9.8%	–10.3%	154.7%
	(2.78%–6.58%)	(6.73%–7.39%)	(7.89%–7.08%)	(2.78%–7.08%)
18–25	79.7%	12.8%	14.8%	213.8%
	(6.22%–11.18%)	(13.81%–15.58%)	(17.00%–19.52%)	(6.22%–19.52%)
26–34	29.2%	29.3%	64.7%	290.3%
	(3.19%–4.12%)	(5.15%–6.66%)	(7.56%–12.45%)	(3.19%–12.45%)
35–49	51.6%	8.7%	43.2%	208.6%
	(2.44%–3.70%)	(4.04%–4.39%)	(5.26%–7.53%)	(2.44%–7.53%)
50+	inf	47.5%	260.4%	inf.
	(0.00%–0.54%)	(0.40%–0.59%)	(1.11%–4.00%)	(0.00–4.00%)

(continued)

Table 3. *(continued)*

	% Change 1994–1998	% Change 1999–2001	% Change 2002–2014	% Change 1994–2014
Education				
Less than high school	−12.7%	6.1%	36.0%	123.9%
	(3.85%–3.36%)	(5.05%–5.36%)	(6.34%–8.62%)	(3.85%–8.62%)
High school	119.4%	28.1%	67.3%	414.5%
	(1.86%–4.08%)	(4.13%–5.29%)	(5.72%–9.57%)	(1.86%–9.57%)
Some college	35.6%	12.0%	40.6%	222.1%
	(3.17%–4.30%)	(5.33%–5.97%)	(7.26%–10.21%)	(3.17%–10.21%)
College graduate	241.5%	13.2%	40.7%	612.2%
	(0.82%–2.80%)	(2.95%–3.34%)	(4.15%–5.84%)	(0.82%–5.84%)
Population				
1 million +	71.1%	14.4%	32.5%	248.0%
	(2.46%–4.21%)	(4.79%–5.48%)	(6.46%–8.56%)	(2.46%–8.56%)
Less than 1 million	73.7%	11.2%	25.3%	229.9%
	(2.51%–4.36%)	(4.92%–5.47%)	(6.61%–8.28%)	(2.51%–8.28%)
Not SMA or CMSA	57.7%	21.4%	55.1%	254.5%
	(1.89%–2.98%)	(3.60%–4.37%)	(4.32%–6.70%)	(1.89%–6.70%)
Total	37.9%	14.2%	38.1%	254.9%
	(2.35%–4.00%)	(4.57%–5.22%)	(6.04%–8.34%)	(2.35%–8.34%)

Source: 1994–2014 NSDUH.

Table 4. Past-Month Hard Drug Use, 1994–2014

	% Change 1994–1998	% Change 1999–2001	% Change 2002–2014	% Change 1994–2014
Sex				
Male	23.9%	43.8%	–22.8%	77.3%
	(0.88%–1.09%)	(1.21%–1.74%)	(2.02%–1.56%)	(0.88%–1.56%)
Female	61.8%	52.7%	–14.0%	135.3%
	(0.34%–0.55%)	(0.55%–0.84%)	(0.93%–0.80%)	(0.34%–0.80%)
Race				
White	44.8%	8.5%	–16.9%	94.8%
	(0.58%–0.84%)	(1.18%–1.28%)	(1.36%–1.13%)	(0.58%–1.13%)
Black	16.9%	25.6%	–50.0%	32.5%
	(0.83%–0.97%)	(0.78%–0.98%)	(2.02%–1.10%)	(0.83%–1.10%)
Hispanic	49.4%	10.2%	0.7%	75.9%
	(0.79%–1.18%)	(1.37%–1.51%)	(1.38%–1.39%)	(0.79%–1.39%)
Age				
12–17	23.4%	–3.3%	–54.4%	–24.1%
	(1.37%–1.69%)	(2.09%–2.02%)	(2.28%–1.04%)	(1.37%–1.04%)
18–25	83.8%	27.1%	–25.1%	89.2%
	(1.48%–2.72%)	(3.28%–4.17%)	(3.74%–2.80%)	(1.48%–2.80%)
26–34	84.3%	14.1%	21.3%	323.5%
	(0.51%–0.94%)	(1.28%–1.46%)	(1.78%–2.16%)	(0.51%–2.16%)
35–49	10.5%	2.1%	–19.6%	94.7%
	(0.57%–0.63%)	(0.94%–0.96%)	(1.38%–1/11%)	(0.57%–1.11%)
50+	–60.0%	12.5%	66.7%	600.0%
	(0.05%–0.02%)	(0.08%–0.09%)	(0.21%–0.35%)	(0.05%–0.35%)

(continued)

Table 4. *(continued)*

	% Change 1994–1998	% Change 1999–2001	% Change 2002–2014	% Change 1994–2014
Education				
Less than high school	39.8%	9.9%	–37.4%	15.9%
	(0.88%–1.23%)	(1.41%–1.55%)	(1.63%–1.02%)	(0.88%–1.02%)
High school	35.2%	48.4%	–14.4%	98.1%
	(0.54%–0.73%)	(0.95%–1.41%)	(1.25%–1.07%)	(0.54%–1.07%)
Some college	5.9%	–1.7%	–7.4%	138.2%
	(0.68%–0.72%)	(1.20%–1.18%)	(1.75%–1.62%)	(0.68%–1.62%)
College graduate	inf.	6.5%	5.5%	inf.
	(0.00%–0.57%)	(0.62%–0.66%)	(0.91%–0.96%)	(0.00%–0.96%)
Population				
1 million +	13.6%	17.3%	–18.6%	67.9%
	(0.81%–0.92%)	(1.33%–1.56%)	(1.67%–1.36%)	(0.81%–1.36%)
Less than 1 million	100.0%	1.7%	–32.9%	108.3%
	(0.48%–0.96%)	(1.17%–1.19%)	(1.49%–1.00%)	(0.48%–1.00%)
Not SMA or CMSA	80.0%	23.5%	–43.8%	54.3%
	(0.35%–0.63%)	(0.68%–0.84%)	(0.96%–0.54%)	(0.35%–0.54%)
Total	45.0%	12.4%	–19.9%	95.0%
	(0.60%–0.87%)	(1.13%–1.27%)	(1.46%–1.17%)	(0.60%–1.17%)

Source: 1994–2014 NSDUH.

as females to report past-month hard drug use and 80 percent more likely to report past-month marijuana use in 2014. Whereas the gender gap in prescription drug misuse narrowed over the past 20 years, the gender gap in marijuana and hard drug use has remained relatively constant over the same period.

Prescription painkiller misuse followed the same basic gendered trends as prescription drug misuse from 1994 to 2014, as shown in Table 5. In 1994, females were twice as likely as males to report past-month prescription painkiller misuse, but by 1998 a slightly higher percentage of males reported past-month prescription painkiller misuse than females. Although males showed a more significant increase in prescription painkiller misuse from 1999 to 2001, females experienced a much more rapid decrease in past-month prescription painkiller misuse (18.8 percent decrease) than males (9.2 percent decrease) from 2002 to 2014. Overall, the increase in past-month prescription painkiller misuse was much more rapid among males than females in the 20-year period between 1994 and 2014. By 2014, males were 28 percent more likely to report past-month prescription painkiller misuse than females.

The gendered pattern of heroin use over the past 20 years, however, has been much different than the gendered patterns of prescription drug misuse. As shown in Table 6, in 1994 males were nearly five times more likely to report past-month heroin use than females, but between 1994 and 1998 males experienced a substantial decrease in past-month heroin use prevalence rates, while females experienced no change in past-month heroin use. By 1998, males were only 33 percent more likely to report past-month heroin use than females. Between 1999 and 2001, past-month heroin use rates among males decreased but increased among females. Even with the increases among males and the decreases among females, however, males remained 50 percent more likely to report past-month heroin use than females in 2001. Between 2002 and 2014, past-month heroin use prevalence rates doubled for males and quadrupled for females. Once again, however, males remained 83 percent more likely to report past-month heroin use than females in 2014. Despite the more rapid increases in heroin use among females over the past 20 years, heroin use continued to be much more prevalent among males than females.

The primary conclusion from the gendered patterns of prescription drug misuse over the past 20 years, especially compared with marijuana and hard drug use patterns, is that prescription drug misuse is *more strongly concentrated among females than males* than other forms of drug use. Note, however, that this does not mean that prescription drug misuse is primarily a female issue; males misuse prescription medications at

Table 5. Past-Month Prescription Painkiller Misuse, 1994–2014

	% Change 1994–1998	% Change 1999–2001	% Change 2002–2014	% Change 1994–2014
Sex				
Male	177.3%	27.5%	–9.2%	704.5%
	(0.22%–0.61%)	(1.20%–1.53%)	(1.95%–1.77%)	(0.22%–1.77%)
Female	125.3%	31.4%	–18.8%	263.2%
	(0.38%–0.48%)	(1.02%–1.34%)	(1.70%–1.38%)	(0.38%–1.38%)
Race				
White	83.9%	28.7%	–20.5%	374.2%
	(0.31%–0.57%)	(1.15%–1.48%)	(1.85%–1.47%)	(0.31%–1.47%)
Black	113.6%	24.5%	31.5%	886.4%
	(0.22%–0.47%)	(1.02%–1.27%)	(1.65%–2.17%)	(0.22%–2.17%)
Hispanic	8.9%	35.1%	–22.7%	277.8%
	(0.45%–0.49%)	(0.94%–1.27%)	(2.20%–1.70%)	(0.45%–1.70%)
Age				
12–17	20.7%	22.3%	–41.0%	98.9%
	(0.87%–1.05%)	(1.88%–2.30%)	(2.93%–1.73%)	(0.87%–1.73%)
18–25	100.0%	41.3%	–38.1%	276.1%
	(0.67%–1.34%)	(2.47%–3.49%)	(4.07%–2.52%)	(0.67%–2.52%)
26–34	58.5%	104.7%	6.0%	541.5%
	(0.41%–0.65%)	(0.85%–1.74%)	(2.48%–2.63%)	(0.41%–2.63%)
35–49	323.1%	19.6%	1.3%	1092.3%
	(0.13%–0.55%)	(1.07%–1.28%)	(1.53%–1.55%)	(0.13%–1.55%)
50+	–100.0%	–23.9%	60.4%	1600.0%
	(0.05%–0.00%)	(0.46%–0.35%)	(0.53%–0.85%)	(0.05%–0.85%)

Education				
Less than high school	0.0%	66.4%	17.4%	252.1%
	(0.73%–0.73%)	(1.19%–1.98%)	(2.19%–2.57%)	(0.73%–2.57%)
High school	168.8%	57.6%	–12.8%	837.5%
	(0.16%–0.43%)	(0.92%–1.45%)	(1.72%–1.50%)	(0.16%–1.50%)
Some college	321.4%	47.5%	–8.7%	1257.1%
	(0.14%–0.59%)	(0.99%–1.46%)	(2.08%–1.90%)	(0.14%–1.90%)
College graduate	237.5%	–41.3%	–7.7%	950.0%
	(0.08%–0.27%)	(1.04%–0.61%)	(0.91%–0.84%)	(0.08%–0.84%)
Population				
1 million +	58.6%	20.3%	–11.6%	451.7%
	(0.29%–0.46%)	(1.23%–1.48%)	(1.81%–1.60%)	(0.29%–1.60%)
Less than 1 million	174.1%	32.1%	–21.8%	496.3%
	(0.27%–0.74%)	(1.06%–1.40%)	(2.06%–1.61%)	(0.27%–1.61%)
Not SMA or CMSA	0.0%	50.5%	–36.2%	156.8%
	(0.37%–0.37%)	(0.91%–1.37%)	(1.49%–0.95%)	(0.37%–0.95%)
Total	80.0%	28.8%	–13.7%	423.3%
	(0.30%–0.54%)	(1.11%–1.43%)	(1.82–1.57%)	(0.30%–1.57%)

Source: 1994–2014 NSDUH.

Table 6. Past-Month Heroin Use, 1994–2014

	% Change 1994–1998	% Change 1999–2001	% Change 2002–2014	% Change 1994–2014
Sex				
Male	–71.4%	–25.0%	100.0%	57.1%
	(0.14%–0.04%)	(0.08%–0.06%)	(0.11%–0.22%)	(0.14%–0.22%)
Female	0.0%	33.3%	300.0%	300.0%
	(0.03%–0.03%)	(0.03%–0.04%)	(0.03%–0.12%)	(0.03%–0.12%)
Race				
White	–55.6%	–20.0%	240.0%	88.9%
	(0.09%–0.04%)	(0.05%–0.04%)	(0.05%–0.17%)	(0.09%–0.17%)
Black	–33.3%	300.0%	66.7%	233.3%
	(0.09%–0.06%)	(0.03%–0.12%)	(0.18%–0.30%)	(0.09%–0.30%)
Hispanic	–62.5%	–60.0%	–8.3%	37.5%
	(0.08%–0.03%)	(0.15%–0.06%)	(0.12%–0.11%)	(0.08%–0.11%)
Age				
12–17	inf.	–78.6%	100.0%	inf.
	(0.00%–0.07%)	(0.14%–0.03%)	(0.03%–0.06%)	(0.00%–0.06%)
18–25	63.6%	75.0%	73.3%	136.4%
	(0.11%–0.18%)	(0.12%–0.21%)	(0.15%–0.26%)	(0.11%–0.26%)
26–34	50.0%	50.0%	614.3%	2400.0%
	(0.02%–0.03%)	(0.04%–0.06%)	(0.07%–0.50%)	(0.02%–0.50%)
35–49	–95.8%	–50.0%	100.0%	–41.7%
	(0.24%–0.01%)	(0.08%–0.04%)	(0.07%–0.14%)	(0.24%–0.14%)
50+	0.0%	0.0%	0.0%	inf.
	(0.00%–0.00%)	(0.00%–0.00%)	(0.06%–0.06%)	(0.00%–0.06%)

Education				
Less than high school	–33.3%	80.0%	52.6%	383.3%
	(0.06%–0.04%)	(0.05%–0.09%)	(0.19%–0.29%)	(0.06%–0.29%)
High school	–87.5%	50.0%	275.0%	–37.5%
	(0.24%–0.03%)	(0.04%–0.06%)	(0.04%–0.15%)	(0.24%–0.15%)
Some college	inf.	–30.0%	166.7%	inf.
	(0.00%–0.08%)	(0.10%–0.07%)	(0.12%–0.32%)	(0.00%–0.32%)
College graduate	0.0%	–50.0%	inf.	inf.
	(0.00%–0.00%)	(0.02%–0.01%)	(0.00%–0.03%)	(0.00%–0.03%)
Population				
1 million +	–81.3%	–10.0%	185.7%	25.0%
	(0.16%–0.03%)	(0.10%–0.09%)	(0.07%–0.20%)	(0.16%–0.20%)
Less than 1 million	133.3%	–50.0%	27.3%	366.7%
	(0.03%–0.07%)	(0.04%–0.02%)	(0.11%–0.14%)	(0.03%–0.14%)
Not SMA or CMSA	0.0%	100.0%	0.0%	inf.
	(0.00%–0.00%)	(0.01%–0.02%)	(0.02%–0.02%)	(0.00%–0.02%)
Total	–50.0%	–16.7%	142.9%	112.5%
	(0.08%–0.04%)	(0.06%–0.05%)	(0.07%–0.17%)	(0.08%–0.17%)

Source: 1994–2014 NSDUH.

a higher rate than females. Rather, the gender gap in prescription drug misuse is much smaller for prescription drug misuse than for marijuana and hard drug use.

Race

Race has also been a central defining feature of prior drug use epidemics. Recall that the crack scare only gained national attention when the use of cocaine entered poor urban minority communities, not when cocaine use was increasing or becoming more dangerous among middle-class white Americans.[2] Do the racial patterns of prescription drug misuse help explain the current public panic about the current prescription drug misuse problem?

Lifetime prevalence rates for prescription drug misuse shown in Table 1 indicate that a greater percentage of white Americans than black or Hispanic Americans have ever misused a prescription medication. Just under a quarter of whites have ever misused a prescription medication, whereas between 14 percent and 15 percent of racial and ethnic minorities have ever misused a prescription medication. The racial gap in prescription drug misuse, however, narrows to irrelevance in the past-year and past-month prevalence rates in the 2014 data. White, black, and Hispanic Americans reported past-year prescription drug misuse at essentially the same rate in 2014, a pattern that is also shown in the past-month prescription drug misuse prevalence rates. Stated simply, white Americans were more likely than black or Hispanic Americans to have misused a prescription medication at some point in their lives, but white Americans were essentially equally as likely as black and Hispanic Americans to report past-year and past-month prescription drug misuse.

The racial dynamics of prescription drug misuse appear to be somewhat different than the racial dynamics with marijuana but similar to the racial patterns for hard drug use. Although the lifetime prevalence rate for marijuana use was higher among white Americans in the 2014 data than black or Hispanic Americans, the past-year and past-month marijuana use data show that black Americans were more likely than whites or Hispanics to report recent use of marijuana. In contrast to the marijuana use data, however, black Americans were less likely to report past-year hard drug use than white or Hispanic Americans, equally likely as white Americans to report past-month hard drug use, and less likely than Hispanic Americans to report past-month hard drug use.

Past-month prescription painkiller misuse is more common among black Americans than white or Hispanic Americans, which means that prescription drug misuse is much more likely to involve prescription painkiller misuse for black Americans than either white or Hispanic Americans. Past-month heroin use, however, is nearly six times more common among white Americans and about four times more likely among Hispanic Americans than black Americans.

A few generalizations can be made about the racial patterns of prescription drug misuse in comparison to patterns of other forms of drug use. First and foremost, the 2014 data clearly show that prescription drug misuse was *not primarily a problem among white Americans*. Second, hard drug use was much more common among white and Hispanic Americans, but marijuana use was more prevalent among black Americans. Third, prescription painkiller misuse was much more prevalent among black Americans than either white or Hispanic Americans, but heroin use is much more of a problem among the white and Hispanic populations in the United States. Taken together, although the data show that prescription drug misuse rates are very similar among all racial and ethnic groups, the choice of opioid to misuse is disproportionately more likely heroin for white and Hispanic Americans and prescription opioids for black Americans.

All types of drug use, however, are less sticky for whites than any other racial and ethnic group. Among the black Americans who have ever misused a prescription medication, 17.9 percent report prescription drug misuse in the past month, but for white Americans who have ever misused a prescription medication, only 10.1 percent report regular use in the past month. The same pattern was shown for marijuana and hard drug use. White Americans, it appears, are much more likely to experiment with all forms of drug use than black Americans, but a higher proportion of white Americans than black Americans avoid becoming regular users of all drugs, including all major categories of misused prescription medications.

Although racial discrepancies in drug use do exist, especially for past-year and past-month marijuana use, the racial disparities in prescription drug misuse are quite small when compared with the racial disparities in the use of marijuana and hard drugs. To illustrate, black Americans were 20 percent more likely to report past-month marijuana use than white Americans in 2014, but black Americans were only 13 percent more likely to report past-month prescription drug misuse in that year, and white and black Americans were equally likely to report past-month hard drug use. In direct contrast to the crack scare, where the emergence of cocaine in black communities in the form of crack created a massive media and political reaction, the prescription drug crisis does not appear to be motivated by any underlying racial or ethnic drug use patterns. Whites misuse prescription medications at the same basic rate as any other racial or ethnic group. As we discuss in later chapters, however, the greater racial equity of prescription drug misuse might be a significant factor defining how the media and politicians have reacted to the crisis.

The racial trends in prescription drug misuse shown in Table 2 are also instructive in understanding the racialized nature of drug use in the United States. In 1994, past-month prescription drug misuse prevalence rates were very similar among white, black, and Hispanic Americans. Between 1994 and 1998, however, the past-month prescription drug misuse rate increased more rapidly among white Americans than among either black or Hispanic Americans. By 1998, white Americans were much more likely to report past-month prescription drug misuse than black or Hispanic Americans. The period between 1999 and 2001 again showed more rapid increases in past-month prescription drug misuse rates among white Americans than black Americans, but Hispanic Americans showed a slight decrease in past-month prescription drug misuse during this period. In 2001, white Americans were again substantially more likely to report past-month prescription drug misuse than black or Hispanic Americans. Strikingly, between 2002 and 2014, white and Hispanic Americans experienced notable decreases in past-month prescription drug misuse prevalence, but black Americans showed a substantial increase in past-month prescription drug misuse. The result of these trends was nearly equal prescription drug misuse prevalence rates among all racial and ethnic groups in 2014. In short, prescription drug misuse was largely concentrated among white Americans in the United States in the early stage of the prescription drug misuse crisis, but prescription drug misuse rates among black Americans have only recently matched and slightly exceeded the prescription drug misuse rates among white Americans.

Racial and ethnic patterns of marijuana and hard drug use shown in Tables 3 and 4 provide a point of reference for better understanding the trends in prescription drug misuse by race. In most years between 1994 and 2014, past-month marijuana use rates were higher among black Americans than either white or Hispanic Americans, but the racial and ethnic gap in marijuana use has narrowed over the past 20 years. In 1994, black Americans were 65 percent more likely to report past-month marijuana use than white Americans and 75 percent more likely to report past-month marijuana use than Hispanic Americans. Because past-month marijuana use rates increased much more rapidly among white and Hispanic Americans than among black Americans between 1994 and 1998, black Americans were only 16 percent more likely to report past-month marijuana use than white Americans and 46 percent more likely to report past-month marijuana use than Hispanic Americans in 1998. Between 1999 and 2001 white Americans experienced further increases in past-month marijuana use rates, but both black and Hispanic Americans showed slight declines in past-month marijuana use rates. By 2001 past-month marijuana use rates were slightly higher among white Americans than black Americans, with the lowest past-month marijuana use rates among Hispanic Americans. The period between 2002 and 2014 showed substantial increases in past-month marijuana use for all racial and ethnic groups. By 2014, black Americans were 20 percent more likely to report past-month marijuana use than whites and 60 percent more likely to report past-month marijuana use than Hispanics. Stated simply, the racial gap in marijuana use has narrowed over the past 20 years.

The racial gap in past-month hard drug use has also narrowed over the past 20 years. In 1994 white Americans were less likely to report past-month hard drug use than black and Hispanic Americans, but between 1994 and 1998 past-month hard drug use rates increased much more rapidly for white and Hispanic Americans than for black Americans. By 1998 Hispanic Americans reported the greatest percentage of past-month hard drug use, followed by black Americans, and white Americans continued to show the lowest hard drug use rate. The black-white gap in hard drug use, however, narrowed between 1994 and 1998. Further increases in past-month hard drug use were shown for all racial and ethnic groups between 1999 and 2001, and by 2001 black Americans showed the lowest past-month hard drug use rate, while Hispanic Americans showed the highest past-month hard drug use rate. Importantly, the black-white gap in hard drug use had reversed by 2001, as white Americans were about 30 percent more likely than black Americans to report past-month hard drug use in that year. Between 2002 and 2014, however, past-month hard drug use prevalence rates decreased for both white and black Americans, but the decrease in hard drug use was much more substantial among black Americans during this period. Hard drug use rates for Hispanic Americans remained steady from 2002 to 2014. The resulting past-month hard drug use rate for black and white Americans was remarkably equal in 2014, but the past-month hard drug use rate for both groups remained higher among Hispanic Americans.

Focusing specifically on the misuse of opiate medications and heroin use by race and ethnicity shown in Tables 5 and 6, substantial increases in both forms of drug use among black Americans from 2002 to 2014 resulted in black Americans being more likely than white or Hispanic Americans to misuse prescription painkillers and heroin in 2014. In 1994 black Americans were less likely than white or Hispanic Americans to misuse prescription painkillers or use heroin, but black Americans experienced a large increase in prescription painkiller misuse between 1994 and 1998, when white and Hispanic Americans experienced smaller increases in past-month painkiller misuse. Further, past-month heroin use rates quadrupled for black Americans between 1999 and 2001 during a period when white and Hispanic Americans experienced notable reductions in heroin use. The rapid increases in both prescription painkiller misuse and heroin use among black Americans over the past 20 years has resulted in black Americans now being more likely than any other racial or ethnic group to misuse opioids, prescriptions, and heroin alike.

Although the data show that opioid misuse, whether it was prescription medication or heroin, quickly became more heavily concentrated among black Americans over the past 20 years, one particular pattern is very important to note—the percentage of white Americans who reported past-month heroin use more than tripled from 2002 to 2014, a period in which heroin use increased much slower or actually declined among other racial or ethnic groups. This substantial increase in past-month heroin use among white Americans coincided with reductions in prescription drug misuse, prescription painkiller misuse, and overall hard drug use during this same period among white Americans. The relationship between heroin use and prescription drug misuse generally and prescription painkiller misuse specifically will be addressed in much more detail in subsequent chapters, but the data certainly indicate that white Americans have been moving away from prescription drug misuse and toward heroin use at a much higher rate than black or Hispanic Americans in recent years.

In sum, the racial and ethnic patterns of prescription drug misuse are complicated. Clearly, black Americans have continued to witness increases in prescription drug misuse in recent years, whereas white and Hispanic Americans have seen decreases in prescription drug misuse during the same recent period between 2002 and 2014, a pattern that also holds for prescription painkiller misuse. Further, the race and ethnic gap in marijuana and hard drug use rates has narrowed over the past 20 years, with black Americans now *less likely* than white and Hispanic Americans to use hard drugs and black Americans are now *more likely* than other groups to misuse prescription medications. The overall conclusion is that black Americans have experienced increases in drug use generally over the past 20 years, but the increase in drug misuse among black Americans has been particularly pronounced in prescription drug and prescription painkiller misuse, especially relative to the drug use patterns of white and

Hispanic Americans. While prescription drug misuse was once heavily concentrated among white Americans, the current data show that this is not the case anymore. That data do show, however, that heroin use has become a much more notable and growing issue among white Americans in recent years than among black and Hispanic Americans.

Age

Prior research has shown drug use to be heavily concentrated among 18- to 34-year-olds in the United States, and the 2014 data shown in Table 1 indicate the same basic pattern holds with prescription drug misuse. With prescription drug misuse, the 18–25, 26–34, and 35–49 age groups showed the highest "ever" misused rates, at about 25 percent on average, in 2014 compared with much smaller percentages of the younger and older groups reporting having ever misused a prescription medication. The 18–25 and 26–34 age groups were also 1.5 to 2 times more likely than older and young groups in the United States to have misused a prescription medication in the past year or past month. The same basic pattern exists by age groups for prescription painkiller misuse and heroin use. For marijuana and hard drug use, however, the prevalence use rates for the 18- to 34-year-old age groups ranged from 2.5 to 7 times higher than the younger and older groups of Americans. Stated simply, a much larger percentage of individuals in the 18–34 age range in the United States than younger and older Americans reported using all types of drugs on a yearly or monthly basis in 2014, but the differences between age groups were smaller for prescription drug misuse than for other drugs.

The stickiness of all drugs decreases with age, including prescription drug misuse, meaning that younger people in the United States who reported having ever used a drug are much more likely than older people to have reported past-month drug use. The high stickiness percentages for the youngest age group in the NSDUH study, the 12–17 age group, likely reflects the simple lack of time to age out of drug use and the relatively low percentage of youths reporting ever having used any of these drugs. The data show that as age increases, increasing numbers of people who have ever experimented with drugs eventually stop using those drugs, including prescription drug misuse. Only a small fraction of the 50+ age group who reported having ever misused a prescription medication also reported past-month prescription drug misuse in 2014.

As shown in Table 2, in 1994 prescription drug misuse was mainly concentrated among young Americans, 25 years of age or younger. Between 1994 and 1998, however, increases in prescription drug misuse were most pronounced in the 18–25 and 35–49 age groups. By 1998, the greatest concentration of prescription drug misusers of any age group by far was the 18–25 age group. Between 1999 and 2001 rapid increases in prescription drug misuse were especially evident in the 26–34 age group, but the 18–25 age group maintained the highest prescription drug misuse rate. From 2002 to 2014 most age groups experienced notable declines in the prevalence of past-month prescription drug misuse, with the most substantial declines shown among the 12–17 age group. The exceptions were the 26–34 and 50+ age groups, which both experienced notable increases in past-month prescription drug misuse rates from 2002 to 2014.

Marijuana use, highlighted in Table 3, followed the same basic trend as prescription drug misuse over the past 20 years, albeit on a much larger scale. The 18–34 age groups were substantially more likely to report past-month marijuana use in each year during the review period than the older and younger age groups. Further, the greatest increases in past-month marijuana use were shown among the 18–34 age groups, especially from 1994 to 1998. By 2014, Americans between the ages of 18 and 26 were approximately two to three times more likely to report past-month marijuana use than the older and younger age groups. Importantly, the 12–17 age group experienced a decrease in marijuana use from 2002 to 2014.

Like prescription drug misuse, the data show that hard drug use was also most strongly concentrated among Americans 25 years of age and younger in 1994, as shown in Table 4. The increases in the prevalence of past-month hard drug use over the subsequent 20 years, however, were more strongly concentrated in the 18–34 age groups, and the 12–17 age group showed notable declines in hard drug use over this period. By 2014 the 18–35 age groups had by far the highest past-month hard drug use rates, more than double the rate of any other age group. Despite having the second-highest past-month hard drug use rate across the first half of the 20-year period investigated, the continued decreases in past-month hard drug use rates over the past 20 years have resulted in the youngest age group now having the second-lowest past-month hard drug use rate, second only to the 50+ age group. Hard drug use shifted away from the youngest Americans and toward the 18–35 age groups over the past 20 years.

Past-month prescription painkiller misuse was also most common among the 12–17 age group in 1994, but as is documented in Table 5, the most rapid increases over the subsequent years were most strongly concentrated among the 18–34 age groups. Americans 25 years of age and younger experienced large declines in past-month prescription drug misuse from 2002 to 2014, but the 26–34 age group experienced an increase in past-month prescription painkiller misuse during that same period. Although the age differences are not as significant for prescription painkiller misuse as was shown for marijuana and hard drug use in 2014, the 18–34 age groups were at least 46 percent more likely to report past-month prescription painkiller misuse than any other age group in 2014.

Heroin use patterns shown in Table 6 by age changed in a more random fashion over the past 20 years. In 1994 heroin use was most common in the 25–49 age group, at 0.2 percent, and next most common in the 18–25 age group, at 0.1 percent. Heroin use was virtually nonexistent in all other age groups in 1994. The 18–25 and 26–34 age groups, however, experienced large increases in past-month heroin use rates across all of the time periods examined over the past 20 years. Past-month heroin use increased an astonishing 614.3 percent between 2002 and 2014 among the 26–34 age group. The result of these heroin use trends over the past 20 years is that the 18–34 age groups showed the strongest concentration of past-month heroin use in 2014, at least double the heroin use rate of all other age groups. Consistent with other drug use trends by age, the 12–17 age group showed the lowest past-month heroin use rate in 2014.

Drug use, regardless of the substance being misused, is most strongly concentrated among the 18–34 age groups, but this has not always been the case. These age groups experienced rapid increases in all forms of drug use over the past 20 years, thereby shifting the prevalence of drug use from the youngest age groups in the United States to the 18–34 age groups. The age gap in drug use, however, is smaller for prescription drug misuse than marijuana or hard drugs. Because future drug use trends are often predicated by drug use patterns among youths, it is instructive that the 12–17 age group has shown substantial declines in most forms of drug use, including prescription drug misuse, in recent years. Young people are using drugs at a lower rate than in the past, which provides some hope that the United States will see declines in drug use rates in the future.

Education

The role of education in drug use processes is complicated by the high rates of drug use shown among college students and by the income disparities associated with the level of education completed. Culturally, however, non–college-educated Americans deserve special attention given the recent discussion of diseases of despair, including prescription drug misuse, that have become evident among noncollege Americans.

The lifetime prevalence rates of all types of drug use, shown in Table 1, were similar by levels of education completed in 2014, with the notable exception that those with some college reported lifetime prevalence drug use rates at slightly higher rates than any other education group. College graduates, although equally likely as high school graduates and high school dropouts to have ever misused a prescription drug, were the least likely to report past-year and past-month prescription drug misuse (past-month prescription drug misuse was about twice as likely among high school dropouts than college graduates). College graduates were also least likely to report past-month marijuana or hard drug use, whereas Americans with some college reported the highest past-month marijuana and hard drug use rates. Involvement in higher education therefore appears to be associated with experimentation with prescription drug misuse and other forms of drug use, but graduating from college makes it less likely that drug use will continue. Drug use therefore was decreasingly sticky with increasing levels of education completed—with the exception that those with some college were more likely than high school graduates and college graduates to continue prescription drug misuse and hard drug use.

We will revisit some issues related to education later in this book, but the main point is that although lifetime prevalence rates are rather uniform across the different levels of education, persistence in using each drug is much more likely for those with lower levels of education completed. The other point, however, is that attending college but not graduating has a unique influence on higher drug use prevalence rates and the continuation of drug use.

As with all other drugs, Americans with a college degree were much less likely to misuse prescription medications than Americans with lesser levels of completed education across the entire time period addressed in the current data. But the education gap in prescription drug misuse, illustrated in Table 2, narrowed dramatically across this time period. In 1994, high school dropouts were 13 times more likely than college graduates to report past-month prescription drug misuse. Because prescription drug misuse rates increased more rapidly among college graduates than among high school dropouts between 1994 and 1998, high school dropouts were only 2.6 times more likely than college graduates to report past-month prescription drug misuse in 1998. From 1999 to 2001, all education groups experienced increases in past-month prescription drug misuse rates except for college graduates, who experienced a 27.5 percent decrease during this period. Minor increases in prescription drug misuse among high school dropouts and increases in prescription drug misuse among all other education groups from 2002 to 2014 resulted in high school dropouts being only twice as likely to report past-month prescription drug misuse as college graduates in 2014. Even with the large increases in prescription drug misuse rates among college graduates over the past 20 years, college graduates remained the least likely education group to report past-month prescription drug misuse in 2014. Americans with some college, however, also experienced major increases in prescription drug misuse rates during this 20-year period and showed the second-highest past-month prescription drug misuse rate in 2014. Prescription drug misuse became a much more popular form of drug abuse among Americans who have been to college, degree or not, over the past 20 years.

Whereas prescription drug misuse increased more slowly among high school graduates than the other education groups over the past 20 years, including a 17.6 percent decrease in past-month prescription drug misuse from 2002 to 2014 (the only group to show a decrease in prescription drug misuse during this period), high school graduates experienced strong and sustained increases in marijuana use during this period. As is illustrated in Table 3, high school graduates and college graduates showed the lowest past-month marijuana use rates in 1994, and although college graduates showed increases in marijuana use in each of the time periods analyzed, high school graduates showed the biggest increases in past-month marijuana use from 1999 to 2001 and from 2002 to 2014. By 2014, high school graduates showed the second highest rate of past-month marijuana use, at 9.6 percent, second only to those with some college education, at 10.2 percent. Interestingly, past-month marijuana use rates among high school dropouts increased at a much lower pace than for any other education group in the United States and actually decreased from 1994 to 1998, when all other education groups showed increases in marijuana use.

Hard drug use followed similar patterns as marijuana and prescription drug misuse over the past 20 years, shown in Table 4, with non–college graduates being more likely to report past-month hard drug use than college graduates across the entire period. Whereas high school graduates experienced a notable increase in past-month hard drug use from 1999 to 2001, when all other education groups showed much lower increases, high school graduates and high school dropouts showed remarkable reductions in past-month hard drug use from 2002 to 2014. Even the "some college" group showed a reduction in past-month hard drug use from 2002 to 2014, although the past-month hard drug use rate for this group remained more than 50 percent higher than for all other education groups in 2014. College graduates, despite maintaining the lowest level of past-month hard drug use of any group in each year over the past 20 years, showed an increase in past-month hard drug use from 2002 to 2014—the only education group to show an increase in hard drug use during this period. Hard drug use, it seems, is becoming more popular among Americans with college degrees.

Trends in opioid misuse over the past 20 years both in prescription painkiller misuse and heroin use, displayed in Tables 5 and 6, also show that Americans with education levels less than a college degree experienced rapid increases in opioid use. While the past-month prescription painkiller misuse rate more than tripled from 1994 to 1998 among college graduates, college graduates showed sizable decreases in prescription painkiller misuse from 1999 to 2001 and from 2002 to 2014. Americans with educations levels below a college degree continued to experience increases in prescription painkiller misuse from 1999 to 2001, but high school graduates and those with some college showed decreases in prescription painkiller misuse from 2002 to 2014. High school dropouts, however, experienced further increases in prescription painkiller misuse from 2002 to 2014, the only education group to show an increase during that period. In contrast, heroin use increased rapidly between 2002 and 2014 for all education groups below a college degree. Importantly, heroin use among college graduates was virtually nonexistent in all years from 1994 to 2014.

As drug use prevalence rates have grown for all groups of Americans over the past 20 years, two important patterns by education level are worth highlighting. First, high school dropouts were the most likely group to use drugs of all forms in 1994, but more rapid increases among high school graduates and those with some college have narrowed the education gap in drug use. In fact, those with some college were more likely than any other education group to use marijuana or hard drugs by 2014 and showed prescription drug misuse rates very close to high school dropouts in the same year, raising questions about the role of drug experimentation in college that contributes to dropping out of college and continuing drug use after college. Second, college graduates were the least likely group to use drugs of any type in 2014, despite rapid increases in prevalence rates in various time periods across the past 20 years. The one area of concern is that college graduates showed evidence of increases in hard drug use from 2002 to 2014 during a period when all other education groups showed decreases in hard drug use. The increase in hard drug use among college-educated Americans, however, was not due to heroin use, as only a tiny fraction of college-educated Americans reported past-month heroin use over the past 20 years.

Rural versus Urban

Perhaps the most compelling story related to prescription drug misuse in the United States is the rural-urban divide. As described in the previous chapter, it is widely believed that prescription drug misuse became a major problem in the United States when OxyContin permeated rural America to treat chronic pain among the aging population of rural laborers, especially in the Appalachian region. The NSDUH includes three categories to capture whether a person lives in a large city (1 million people or larger), a smaller city (fewer than 1 million people), or a city that it is not located within a metropolitan statistical area. The latter category best approximates living in a rural area. Cities that are part of a metropolitan statistical area, regardless of size, are considered urban.

Although many Americans perceive prescription drug misuse to be primarily a problem in rural areas, the 2014 data displayed in Table 1 shows that rural areas had lower prevalence rates for all forms of drug use, including prescription drug misuse, than urban areas. The lifetime prescription drug misuse prevalence rate in urban areas was just over 20 percent in 2014, whereas the lifetime prevalence rate of prescription drug misuse in rural locations was 15 percent. The same pattern was shown for both past-year and past-month prescription drug misuse rates—prescription drug misuse was simply more prevalent in urban areas than in rural areas in 2014. Drug use, including prescription drug misuse, was also slightly more sticky in large urban cities than in smaller urban areas and rural locations. In short, rural areas do not appear to have a unique problem with prescription drug misuse or any other form of drug use. As with the other demographic factors examined in this chapter, however, prescription drug use was more of a problem in rural areas than in urban areas compared with other drugs. For instance, prescription drug misuse was 1.5 times more likely in large urban cities than in rural areas in 2014, but hard drug use was 2.5 times more likely in large urban cities than in rural areas. Similarly, prescription painkiller misuse was 1.7 times more likely in large urban cities than in rural areas in 2014, but heroin use was 10 times more prevalent in large cities than in rural areas.

The problems associated with prescription drug misuse in rural areas have been well documented in academic and media sources, and although the 2014 data did not show that prescription drug misuse is heavily concentrated in rural areas, did prescription drug misuse in rural areas grow faster than prescription drug misuse in urban areas? The answer is no. As shown in Table 2, rural residents in the United States were about 1.2 times more likely to report past-month prescription drug misuse than residents of large metropolitan cities in 1994. The combination of increases in prescription drug misuse in urban cities and declines in prescription drug misuse in rural areas, however, resulted in residents of urban areas being much more likely to report past-month prescription drug misuse than residents in rural areas by 2014. Except for a larger increase in the past-month prevalence rate for prescription drug misuse in rural areas from 1999 to 2001 than was shown in urban cities, prescription drug misuse rates in rural areas either decreased when the same rates in urban cities increased or decreased faster than was shown in urban cities in the other time periods over the past 20 years. Data from the past 20 years therefore show that rural areas did not experience a more significant problem with prescription drug misuse than urban areas.

In comparison, the increase in marijuana use over the past 20 years shown in Table 3 was relatively even between rural and urban areas. Urban areas have consistently shown higher past-month marijuana use rates than rural areas, with marijuana prevalence rates being approximately 25 percent greater in urban areas than rural areas over the past 20 years. Similarly, hard drug use patterns over the past 20 years reveal that the changes in hard drug use have been similar in rural areas as in urban areas. Like prescription drug misuse patterns, however, hard drug use, shown in Table 4, did increase more rapidly in rural areas from 1999 to 2001 than in urban areas, but the decreases in hard drug use were much more notable in rural areas from 2002 to 2014 than in urban areas. Simply stated, the data show that there was a unique but minor spike in both prescription drug misuse and hard drug use from 1999 to 2001 in rural areas that quickly subsided between 2002 and 2014.

The pattern of drug use increasing rapidly from 1999 to 2001 but dropping quickly thereafter was also shown in prevalence rate patterns for past-month prescription painkiller misuse, illustrated in Table 5. Prescription painkiller misuse was slightly more common in rural areas than urban areas in 1994, and prescription painkiller misuse increased more rapidly in rural areas from 1999 to 2001. The greatest declines in prescription painkiller misuse, however, were shown in rural areas from 2002 to 2014. Prescription painkiller misuse, once a slightly more common problem in rural areas than in urban areas, was 68 percent more likely in urban areas by 2014.

Heroin use prevalence rates, documented in Table 6, were extremely low in rural areas over the past 20 years, showing only minor changes across the periods. The most striking pattern in heroin use prevalence rates over the past 20 years is the large increase in past-month heroin use in major metropolitan areas from 2002 to 2014, with heroin use in major urban areas nearly tripling during this period. Rural areas, however, did not have a heroin use problem compared with urban areas, with major metropolitan areas showing past-month heroin use rates 10 times higher than rural areas. Heroin, it seems, is also an urban problem.

Taken together, with the exception of higher initial rates of prescription drug misuse in 1994, primarily in the form of prescription painkiller misuse, and more rapid increases in prescription drug misuse from 1999 to 2001, rural areas have not experienced a faster-growing problem with prescription drug misuse than urban areas over the past 20 years. Rural areas in the United States do not have a unique prescription drug misuse problem.

Summary of the Demographic Patterns of Drug Use

Overall, all forms of drug use increased in the periods between 1994 and 2001 except for heroin use, which decreased during these periods, and prescription drug misuse increased faster than other forms of drug use. Between 2002 and 2014, however, drug use generally declined, especially prescription drug misuse. The primary exception to this pattern is marijuana use, which continued to increase between 2002 and 2014. More disturbingly, heroin use has recently increased dramatically in the United States.

Although no group of Americans has been immune to the growth in drug use generally or prescription drug misuse specifically over the past 20 years, a few generalizations related to the demographic trends in drug use are worth noting. First, in the mid-1990s, prescription drug misuse was more common among some groups that are not generally known to be frequent drug users. For instance, females were more likely than males to report past-month prescription drug misuse, white Americans were more likely than black Americans to report past-month prescription drug misuse, and rural residents were more likely than urban residents were in 1994 to report past-month prescription drug misuse. Because the same patterns were not shown for any other form of drug use, it is clear that prescription drug misuse was a unique problem among groups not typically viewed as being common drug users in the United States in the early stages of the prescription drug misuse problem. But the data suggest that more typical drug users (i.e., males, urban residents, and black Americans) quickly caught on to the prescription drug misuse fad that began among nontraditional drug using groups. By 1998, males and residents of urban areas reported higher past-month prescription drug misuse rates than females and rural residents, respectively. The race gap in prescription drug misuse, however, narrowed more slowly, with prescription drug misuse rates among black Americans surpassing the prescription drug misuse rates of white Americans much more recently.

Despite the traditional demographic patterns of drug use emerging more recently for prescription drug misuse, it must also be noted that the gender, race, and urban-rural gap remains much narrower for prescription drug misuse than other forms of drug use. In 2014, for instance, males were only 10 percent more likely to report past-month prescription drug misuse than females, but in the same year, males were 80 percent more likely to report past-month marijuana use and 95 percent more likely to report past-month hard drug use than females. Although prescription drug misuse is not *primarily* a white, female, and/or rural problem in the United States, prescription drug misuse is *more of a problem* among whites, females, and/or rural residents than other forms of drug use. The weaker demographic concentrations for prescription drug misuse stand in stark contrast to prior drug scares and provide evidence for why the public and politicians have been strongly focused on public health solutions for the prescription drug problem in the United States—a stark contrast from the criminal justice solutions associated with past drug scares.

The national data over the past 20 years, however, offer glimpses of hope for a lessening of the prescription drug misuse problem in the United States. The youngest group of Americans, for instance, have shown unmistakable declines in prescription drug misuse in recent years, greater reductions than any other age group. Youths also showed major reductions in hard drug use in recent years and lesser magnitude reductions in marijuana use. To the degree that drug abuse patterns among youths in the United States are predictive of future drug abuse trends in the country more broadly, the United States will likely see further reductions in prescription drug misuse as current youths age into adulthood in future years.

The cyclical nature of drug abuse in the United States, however, also holds dire warnings for the future of drug abuse in the United States. Just as prescription painkiller misuse has declined rapidly among youths in recent years, heroin use has increased dramatically among this group. The connection between prescription painkiller misuse and heroin use will be examined in more detail later in the book, but the dramatic increases in heroin use among females, white Americans, urban residents, and all Americans below 50 years of age suggest that heroin use might very well be the next drug abuse fad in the United States.

With only 2.3 percent of Americans currently reporting past-month prescription drug misuse, it is important to question whether the United

States is currently experiencing a prescription drug misuse *epidemic*. Before we address that question, it is important to examine whether the growth in prescription drug misuse was due to new drug users attracted solely to prescription drugs or due to existing drug users adding prescription medications to their drug use repertoires.

Are Prescription Drug Misusers New Drug Users?

The demographic trends in prescription drug misuse suggest that groups (i.e., females, whites, rural residents) not normally associated with drug use are misusing prescription medications at a disproportionately higher rate than other drugs. The question that we address next is whether the rapid growth in prescription drug misuse included new drug users or whether the increase in prescription drug misuse was largely concentrated among people who were already drug users. Stated simply, do prescription drugs attract people already predisposed to other forms of drug use, or did prescription drug misuse develop among Americans who were not using other forms of illicit drugs?

To answer this question, we once again turn to the NSDUH data for answers. Because this is not a simple question to answer with national data, we use several different strategies to provide evidence. First, we need to start by explaining that the prevalence of overall drug use increased from 1994 to 1998 by 60.6 percent, from 1999 to 2011 by 14.2 percent, and from 2002 to 2014 by 24.6 percent. Given the large percentage increases in drug use in each period as well as the large percentage increases in prescription drug misuse noted above from 1994–1998 and from 1999–2001, it would be easy to assume that prescription drug misuse accounted for the vast majority of the increase in overall prevalence of drug use in these periods. This assumption, however, is likely incorrect, as marijuana use and hard drug use also increased across these same periods. A more accurate assessment of the degree to which prescription drug misuse influenced overall drug use patterns is needed.

We start our investigation by determining the degree to which prescription drug misuse was a part of overall drug use patterns at different periods over the past 20 years. The logic is that if the percentage of overall drug use that included prescription drug misuse increased in any given period, that is evidence that prescription drug misuse became a more significant aspect of overall drug use in that period and that increases in overall drug use were at least in part due to new drug users who misused prescription medications in that period. The results, shown in Table 7, indicate that the percentage of all drug use that included prescription drug misuse

Table 7. Increase in Drug Use Due to Type of Drug

	1994–1998	1999–2001	2002–2014
Any drug use	60.6% (2.97%–4.77%) **1.80**	14.2% (5.93%–6.77%) **0.84**	24.6% (8.08%–10.07%) **1.99**
Marijuana use	37.9% (2.35%–4.00%) **1.65**	14.2% (4.57%–5.22%) **0.65**	38.1% (6.04%–8.34%) **2.30**
Prescription drug misuse	55.1% (0.49%–0.76%) **0.27**	20.7% (1.64%–1.98%) **0.34**	–10.1% (2.58%–2.32%) **–0.26**
Hard drug use	45.0% (0.60%–0.87%) **0.27**	12.4% (1.13%–1.27%) **0.14**	–19.9% (1.46%–1.17%) **–0.29**
% Drug users who use marijuana	6.0% (79.12%–83.86%) **4.74**	0.0% (77.07%–77.10%) **0.03**	10.8% (74.75%–82.82%) **8.07**
% Drug users who abuse prescription drugs	–3.5% (16.50%–15.93%) **–0.57**	5.7% (27.66%–29.25%) **1.59**	–27.8% (31.93%–23.04%) **–8.89**
% Drug users who use hard drugs	–9.7% (20.20%–18.24%) **–1.96**	–1.6% (19.06%–18.76%) **–0.3**	–35.7% (18.07%–11.62%) **–6.45**
% Increase in drug use b/c marijuana	91.7%	77.4%	115.6%
% Increase in drug use b/c prescription drugs	15.0%	40.5%	–13.1%
% Increase in drug use b/c hard drugs	15.0%	16.7%	–14.6%

Source: 1994–2014 NSDUH.

decreased slightly from 1994 to 1998, increased slightly from 1999 to 2001, and dramatically decreased from 2002 to 2014. Prescription drug misuse therefore did attract new drug users for a short period of time from 1999 to 2001. The findings also show that prescription drug misuse fell out of favor in the United States and that marijuana gained in popularity from 2002 to 2014. Importantly, the percentage of all drug use that included hard drug use decreased in each of the three periods, thereby indicating that hard drug use is becoming less common among drug users in the United States. The data also raise the possibility that some hard drug users turned away from hard drugs and toward prescription drug misuse, especially in the 1999–2001 period.

To better describe the degree to which prescription drug misuse influenced overall drug use trends in the United States over the past 20 years, we begin by calculating the raw population percentage changes in past-month drug use in each of the three periods. In short, the raw population percentage changes shown in Table 7 in boldface represent the increase or decrease in proportion of the population that reported past-month drug use over that period. To illustrate what these percentages mean, by 1998, 0.27 percent more of the U.S. population reported past-month prescription drug misuse than in 1994. Across that same period, 1.80 percent more Americans reported past-month drug use of any type in 1998 compared with 1994. Using these numbers, we calculate that 15 percent of the overall increase in drug use from 1994 to 1998 was due to prescription drug misuse (0.27 percent/1.80 percent = 15 percent). In contrast, 91.7 percent of the increase in overall drug use from 1994 to 1998 was due to marijuana use. Americans who started using drugs between 1994 and 1998 were therefore much more likely to use marijuana than misuse prescription medications. Between 1999 and 2001, however, prescription drug misuse accounted for 40.5 percent of the increase in overall drug use, and marijuana use accounted for only 77.4 percent of the increase in overall drug use. Because overall drug use continued to increase from 2002 to 2014 while prescription drug misuse decreased, the data show that the increases in marijuana use during this period accounted for more than 100 percent of the increase in overall drug use. This means that new drug users during this period were overwhelmingly likely to choose marijuana and that a sizable number of prescription drug misusers and hard drug users moved to marijuana.

Prescription drug misuse therefore became a much more significant aspect of overall drug use between 1999 and 2001, but the overwhelming majority of new drug users over the past 20 years used marijuana. A discerning reader, however, will notice that the percentage increases in the overall prevalence of past-month prescription drug attributed to each category of drug use does not add to 100 percent. This is because drug users will often abuse more than one type of drug on a regular basis. The next step in understanding the role of prescription drug misuse in determining overall drug use trends in each period is therefore to examine trends in polydrug use (i.e., using more than one drug) across each period. To accomplish this analysis, we created mutually exclusive categories of drug use (marijuana only, hard drugs only, prescription drugs only, and prescription drugs and other drugs) and tracked these trends over each period. The main evidence for whether the expansion of prescription drug misuse was new drug users or whether the expansion occurred among existing drug users is shown in the differences in trends over time in marijuana-only, prescription-only users, and polydrug users who also misuse prescription medications. The logic is that if marijuana-only and hard drug–only use population proportions decreased over time but prescription and other drug use proportions increased, this is evidence that those who were using marijuana or hard drugs had simply added prescription drugs to their drug use repertoires. This finding would reject that the drug use increases over the past 20 years were due to new prescription drug misusers. On the other hand, if the prescription-only group increased over time while the marijuana-only or hard drug–only groups remained steady or increased, this would be evidence that prescription drug misuse did indeed attract new drug users.

The results in Table 8 show that the vast majority, or 75 percent, of the overall drug use increase between 1994 and 1998 was due to increases in marijuana-only use and that an additional 10.6 percent of the increase in overall drug use was due to the increase in marijuana and hard drug use. Only 8.3 percent of the increase in overall drug use during this period was due to prescription drug misuse only, and an additional 1.1 percent of the increase was accounted for by marijuana and prescription drug misuse. Additionally, only 4.4 percent of the overall increase in drug abuse from 1994 to 1998 was due to increases in the use of all three categories of drugs. Prescription drugs, however, became a more significant aspect of the increase in overall drug use between 1999 and 2001, whereas marijuana became less important during this period. From 1999 to 2001, 52.4 percent of the increase in overall drug use was due to increases in marijuana-only use, and only 3.6 percent of the increase was due to marijuana and hard drug use over this period. On the other hand, 17.9 percent of the increase in overall drug use from 1999 to 2001 was due to increases in prescription drug misuse only, and 13.1 percent of the increase was due to marijuana and prescription drug misuse increases. An additional 8.3 percent of the

Table 8. Increase in Drug Use Due to Polydrug Use

	% Change 1994–1998	% Change 1999–2001	% Change 2002–2014
Any drug use	60.6% (2.97%–4.77%) **1.80**	14.2% (5.93%–6.77%) **0.84**	24.6% (8.08%–10.07%) **1.99**
PDM, marijuana, and hard drug use	266.7% (0.03%–0.11%) **0.08**	31.8% (0.22%–0.29%) **0.07**	–20.7% (0.29%–0.23%) **–0.06**
PDM and marijuana use	12.5% (0.16%–0.18%) **0.02**	27.5% (0.40%–0.51%) **0.11**	–3.9% (0.76%–0.73%) **–0.03**
Marijuana and hard drug use	79.2% (0.24%–0.43%) **0.19**	6.1% (0.49%–0.52%) **0.03**	–12.7% (0.55%–0.48%) **–0.07**
PDM and hard drug use	0.0% (0.04%–0.04%) **0.00**	0.0% (0.09%–0.09%) **0.00**	–20.0% (0.10%–0.08%) **–0.02**
Marijuana use only	69.9% (1.93%–3.28%) **1.35**	12.7% (3.46%–3.90%) **0.44**	55.8% (4.43%–6.90%) **2.47**
PDM only	51.7% (0.29%–0.44%) **0.15**	16.0% (0.94%–1.09%) **0.15**	–10.5% (1.43%–1.28%) **–0.15**

(continued)

Table 8. *(continued)*

	% Change 1994–1998	% Change 1999–2001	% Change 2002–2014
Hard drug use only	85.7% (0.21%–0.30%) **0.09**	12.1% (0.33%–0.37%) **0.04**	–27.5% (0.51%–0.37%) **–0.14**
% Increase in drug use b/c PDM, marijuana, and hard drug use	4.4%	8.3%	–3.0%
% Increase in drug use b/c PDM and marijuana use	1.1%	13.1%	–1.5%
% Increase in drug use b/c marijuana and hard drug use	10.6%	3.6%	–3.5%
% Increase in drug use b/c PDM and hard drug use	0.0%	0.0%	–1.0%
% Increase in drug use b/c marijuana use only	75.0%	52.4%	124.1%
% Increase in drug use b/c PDM only	8.3%	17.9%	–7.5%
% Increase in drug use b/c hard drug use only	5.0%	4.8%	–7.0%

Source: 1994–2014 NSDUH.

increase in overall drug use during this period was due to the use of all three categories of drugs.

Because the population proportions of marijuana-only and hard drug–only use increased during both the 1994–1998 and 1999–2001 periods and because the prescription drug–only misuse population proportions also increased during the same periods, it appears that prescription drug misuse did indeed attract new drug users during this period. It is important to note that these new drug users were very unlikely to use hard drugs along with prescription medication misuse.

The period between 2002 and 2014 was marked by continued increases in marijuana use but a decrease in prescription drug misuse and hard drug use. Because the population proportions of prescription drug–only and marijuana and prescription drug misuse decreased but marijuana-only drug use patterns increased, the 2002–2014 period likely marked a movement away from prescription drug misuse and toward marijuana-only use. The proportion of the population who reported past-month drug use of any type increased by 1.99 percent from 2002 to 2014, but 2.47 percent more of the population reported past-month marijuana-only use from 2002 to 2014. This means that marijuana-only use accounted for 124.1 percent of the increase in overall drug use from 2002 to 2014 and also means that all other patterns of drug use combinations decreased in population proportions over this period. As Americans moved away from prescription drug misuse and to a lesser extent hard drug use, Americans moved rapidly toward marijuana-only use during this period.

Prescription drug use clearly attracted a meaningful number of new drug users during the early years of the prescription drug problem in the United States, but drug use patterns have shifted in recent years away from prescription drug misuse and toward marijuana again. The effect of public policies designed to deter prescription drug misuse will be examined in detail later in the book, but the national data from 2002–2014 suggests that Americans' minds are being changed about the attractiveness of prescription drug misuse in relation to marijuana.

A Prescription Drug Misuse Epidemic?

Taken together, the drug use prevalence data over the past 20 years provide some valuable information that helps us better understand the scale, scope, and development of the prescription drug misuse problem in the United States. First, the most recent information available shows that 1 out of every 5 Americans ages 12 and older has misused a prescription medication at least once in their lifetimes, 1 out of every 18 Americans has misused a prescription medication in the past year, and 1 out of every 43 Americans have misused a prescription medication in the past month. Despite recent prescription drug misuse declines in the United States, prescription drug misuse remains second in prevalence only to marijuana use.

Another notable finding thus far is that the demographic patterns of prescription drug misuse are different than the demographic patterns of other forms of drug use. Like marijuana and hard drug use, males are now more likely than females to misuse prescription medications, white Americans are less likely than black Americans to misuse prescription medications, and urban residents are more likely than rural residents to misuse prescription medications. The difference between prescription drug misuse and other forms of drug use, however, is in the magnitude of the demographic differences. The gender, race, and rural-urban gaps in prescription drug misuse are much narrower than the same gaps in marijuana and hard drug use. Stated simply, prescription drug misuse is *more of a problem* among the demographic groups not historically implicated in prior drug scares and the demographic groups more likely to use marijuana and/or hard drugs. The issue of income in prescription drug use patterns will be examined in detail in a subsequent chapter, as prescription drug misuse has been framed in media portrayals as a middle-class problem, but at this point it is clear that the demographic patterns of prescription drug misuse are different than other forms of drug use.

Prescription drug misuse is clearly a problem in the United States that, despite recent reductions in prevalence, has grown over the past 20 years. The question that remains, however, is whether prescription drug misuse reached epidemic levels in the United States. The answer to this question is quite complex and depends on the definition of the term "epidemic." The term "epidemic" is widely misused to refer to any issue that appears to be a problem in a society and needs urgent attention. The term "epidemic," however, was developed by epidemiologists to explain the emergence and rise in disease, not drug use. Historically, the term "epidemic" was primarily used to describe the outbreak of a life-threatening infectious diseases that created elevated mortality rates in a population. In the 19th century, a number of epidemics were reported in the United States that related to outbreaks of yellow fever, cholera, and other infectious diseases. Because prior epidemics were often associated with increased mortality, epidemics generally created great fear in the population. More recently, the term "epidemic" has been used loosely to describe chronic conditions that are not necessarily associated with increased mortality.

The mass media often uses the term "epidemic" to describe patterns of behavior that are inconsistent with the CDC's definition. The U.S. population has become weary of the term.

National data indicate that fluctuations in the prevalence of substance use are common. Elected officials and the media, however, are quick to label substance use at any level an epidemic. In recent history we have seen several so-called drug epidemics in the United States, including heroin use in the 1960s, marijuana use in the 1970s, crack in the 1980s, and ecstasy and methamphetamine in the 1990s. Prescription drug misuse emerged as an epidemic in media and political discourse in the 2000s.

It is important to note, however, that these so-called drug epidemics often do not fit the CDC's definition of an epidemic. An example of this can be found in the drug methamphetamine, a drug that has been around since the 1930s but wasn't recognized as a problem drug until the 1960s. There is a long history of drugs being tied to marginalized groups as a way to frame them as a danger to society. This includes opium being linked to Chinese immigrants, cocaine being linked to freed slaves in the U.S. South, and marijuana being linked to Mexican immigrants in the Southwest. For methamphetamine, it was outlaw biker gangs who manufactured and sold the drug and gay men who used it. In the 1990s, methamphetamine became the number one drug threat even though data from the NSDUH indicated that less than 5 percent of the population reported use of methamphetamine. The media, however, promoted fear that methamphetamine that was ravaging the country, leaving many communities in complete chaos. This rhetoric was not matched by reality, as methamphetamine accounted for a relatively small proportion of the overall drug problems in the United States.

The CDC defines an epidemic as "an increase, often sudden, in the number of cases of a disease above what is normally expected in that population in that area."[3] Assuming that drug use can be equated to infectious diseases, to determine whether the prescription drug misuse crisis in the United States is an epidemic, we must be able to define a normal level of prescription drug misuse in the country. Defining a normal level of prescription drug misuse, however, is problematic in and of itself. In a culture based on "Just Say No" and zero tolerance, any level of substance use is defined as problematic. So, instead of defining a drug epidemic as something that occurs when the prevalence of substance use exceeds an expected level of use, the term "epidemic" is often used to describe any level of drug use, but expecting zero substance use in a society is unrealistic. Because the term "epidemic" is used to communicate fear and panic in a time of crisis, which often leads to restrictive and punitive public responses, describing any drug use pattern as an epidemic in the United States is highly problematic. The use of the term also stigmatizes drug users and makes it difficult to identify the reasons why drug use has increased and to identify the best ways to reduce the harms associated with drug use.

That said, it is important to consider the prevalence of prescription drug misuse in the United States as well as the documented increases in prescription drug over the past 20 years in determining whether the term "epidemic" should be used to describe the prescription drug misuse problem in the country. Although there are many ways to define the endemic level of drug use in a culture, the remarkable stability in past-month prescription drug misuse and hard drug use from 1994 to 1998 provides a starting point for understanding normal levels of drug use in our current culture. Between 1994 and 1998, both past-month prescription drug misuse and past-month hard drug use hoovered just below 1 percent of the population, which suggests that the normal endemic level of prescription drug misuse would be at about 1 percent of the population. Although the methodology for collecting information about drug use had changed by 2002, the prevalence of past-month prescription drug misuse was quite steady at around 2.5–2.6 percent of the U.S. population between 2002 and 2014. Prescription drug misuse rates apparently tripled over this period. A tripling in the rate of any form of drug use is certainly in line with the definition of an epidemic.

As described throughout this chapter, however, the NSDUH changed data-collection methodologies in 1999 and 2002. These changes, namely the implementation of a computer-aided survey and a small amount of compensation for completing the survey, were designed to allow the respondents to more freely admit drug use and encouraged more people to complete the survey. The apparent tripling of past-month prescription drug misuse rates are therefore quite possibly the result of methodological changes, not necessarily increases in prescription drug misuse. Because the comparable surveys from 1994–1998 and 1999–2001 both show increases in prescription drug misuse, however, prescription drug misuse has definitely increased over the past 20 years, but the scale of the increase is likely much less than the data appear to show at first glance.

Focusing just on the period between 2002 and 2014, a period in which the data-collection methodology by the NSDUH was consistent and the results are comparable between years, the lowest prevalence rate for prescription drug misuse was 2.25 percent in 2011, and the highest prevalence rate was 2.69 percent in 2009. The criticisms of using the term "epidemic" to describe drug use in the United States notwithstanding, in sheer numbers alone, any drug use pattern with less than 3 percent past-month prevalence rates is difficult to describe as an epidemic. This is especially true when the most recent data show steady or declining prevalence rates for prescription drug misuse during the most recent period.

Given all of these factors, people who study both drug use crises and traditional disease epidemics will disagree in good faith about whether the current prescription drug misuse problem should be defined as an epidemic. Certainly, prescription drug misuse in the United States is a problem in urgent need of public attention. Given the relatively low past-month prescription drug misuse prevalence rates and the relatively modest increases in prescription drug misuse rates over the comparable periods during the past 20 years, however, prescription drug *misuse* does not meet the definition of an epidemic in epidemiological terms. In contrast, prescription drug misuse *deaths* might provide more insight into the question as to whether the United States is experiencing a prescription drug epidemic, the topic to which we turn in the next section.

The Prescription Drug Misuse Death Epidemic

Media and politicians present the prescription drug misuse problem in the United States as a crisis in need of urgent public attention. Despite the claim above that prescription drug *misuse* has likely not reached levels to be considered an epidemic, it is quite possible that the media and politicians are absolutely correct that the United States is experiencing a prescription drug misuse *death* epidemic. The vast majority of media stories and political messages about the prescription drug misuse problem in the United States focus on deaths, near deaths, or growing death rates attributed to prescription drug misuse. The media and politicians almost never mention *actual rates of prescription drug misuse* in the United States. As described in the previous section, past-month prevalence use rates for prescription drug misuse are quite small (less than 3 percent), and the growth in prescription drug misuse over the past 20 years has been noticeable but modest, with the most recent period showing declines in prescription drug misuse rates. Further, no specific demographic group has experienced prescription drug misuse prevalence rates or increases over the past 20 years that have been so significant as to reach epidemic levels.

In the following section, we use the CDC Wonder database to investigate whether the United States is actually experiencing a prescription drug misuse *death* epidemic. The CDC Wonder database includes the underlying cause of death reported on every death certificate in the United States each year since 1999. At the time of this writing data were available up to 2015, but because we make comparisons between the trends shown in the NSDUH data that was only available up to 2014, comparisons between prescription drug misuse rates and prescription drug misuse death rates focus on the period between 1999 and 2014.

Prescription Drug Misuse Death Rates in the United States

In 2015, the most recent data available at the time of the writing, 52,404 people died from a drug overdose, for a rate of 16.2 people per 100,000. Prescription medication misuse alone caused 29,728 overdose deaths in 2015, accounting for 56.7 percent of all drug overdose deaths, for an overdose death rate of 9.2 people per 100,000. Prescription drugs were in fact associated with more overdose deaths than all the traditional illicit drugs combined. Heroin, cocaine, cannabis, LSD, other hallucinogens, and psychostimulants with abuse potential (mostly methamphetamine) were responsible for 21,823 overdose deaths in 2015, for a rate of 6.8 overdose deaths per 100,000. In comparison to other common causes of death, drug overdoses accounted for more deaths than traffic accidents (35,092 deaths), suicide (44,193 deaths), and homicide (15,872 deaths) in 2015. Prescription drugs alone accounted for nearly as many deaths as traffic accidents in 2015 and killed double the number of Americans as did homicides. In the context of unintentional deaths, drug overdoses generally and prescription drug overdoses specifically are a major problem in the United States.

Of the 29,728 prescription drug overdose deaths in 2015, 22,598 were attributed to prescription opioid medication accidental overdoses, meaning that 43.1 percent of all accidental drug overdoses in the United States involved a prescription opioid overdose and that 73.4 percent of all prescription drug involved overdose deaths. To put this information in context, more Americans were killed by a prescription opioid alone than from homicide in 2015. Heroin, in contrast, was responsible for 12,989 overdose deaths in 2015, far fewer deaths than were caused by prescription drug misuse generally or prescription opioid misuse specifically. In 2015 there were a total of 33,091 opioid overdose deaths combined, including deaths from prescription opioids, heroin, and synthetic opioids (primarily fentanyl). Opioids, whether in the form of prescription drugs or an illicit drug (heroin, synthetics), accounted for 63.1 percent of all accidental drug overdose deaths in 2015. Accidental overdose deaths from prescription drug misuse, primarily prescription opioid misuse, are clearly a major problem in the United States.

Trends in Prescription Drug Misuse Deaths

Prescription drug misuse death rates have also increased substantially since 1999. As shown in Table 9, 2.7 per 100,000 Americans died from an accidental prescription drug overdose in 1999. By 2001, the prescription drug misuse accidental overdose rate increased to 3.2 per 100,000 Americans, an increase of 18.5 percent from 1999. Between 2002 and 2014, the prescription drug misuse overdose death rate increased from 4 to 8.1 per 100,000 Americans, an increase of 102.5 percent. Recall that the past-month prescription drug misuse rate in the United States reported in the NSDUH increased by 20.7 percent between 1999 and 2001 and decreased by 10.1 percent from 2002 to 2014. When the past-month prescription drug misuse rates are compared with changes in the prescription drug misuse overdose death rates from the same periods, it is clear that prescription drug misuse death rates have grown much faster than the prescription drug misuse rates in the United States. The prescription drug misuse overdose death rate tripled between 1999 and 2014, and even under the most generous assumption that the methodological changes by the NSDUH in 2002 had no influence on the population estimates for prescription drug misuse during this period, the percentage of the population who reported past-month prescription drug misuse only doubled during this same period. It is therefore clear that the prescription drug misuse *death* crisis has grown much faster than the prescription drug *misuse* crisis in the United States, especially between 2002 and 2014.

Because death statistics are provided on a yearly basis in the CDC Wonder system, comparisons with past-year prescription drug misuse prevalence rates and death rates are more accurate. As illustrated in Table 9, between 1999 and 2001, the percentage of the U.S. population who reported past-year prescription drug misuse increased by 21.6 percent, which is a faster growth rate than the 18.5 percent increase in prescription drug misuse deaths during this same period. From 2002 to 2014, however, past-year prescription drug misuse decreased by 11.3 percent, but the death rate from accidental prescription drug overdoses increased by 102.5 percent. Clearly, the deadliness of prescription drug misuse has increased substantially in recent years. *As prescription drug misuse prevalence rates decreased, the prescription drug misuse overdose death rate more than doubled.* Stated simply, prescription drug misuse has become more deadly.

Table 9. Prescription Drug Misuse and Deaths, 1999–2014

	% Change PDM Death Rate 1999–2001	% Change Past-Year PDM Use 1999–2001	% Change PDM Death Rate 2002–2014	% Change Past-Year PDM Use 2002–2004	% Change PDM Death Rate 1999–2014
Sex					
Male	–12.12%	23.69%	70.83%	–9.32%	148.48%
	(3.3–2.9)	(4.01%–4.96%)	(4.8–8.2)	(6.44%–5.84%)	(3.3–8.2)
Female	23.81%	19.68%	109.09%	–13.18%	228.57%
	(2.1–2.6)	(3.76%–4.50%)	(3.3–6.9)	(5.84%–5.07%)	(2.1–6.9)
Race					
White	38.71%	25.86%	118.37%	–13.31%	245.16%
	(3.1–4.3)	(4.06%–5.11%)	(4.9–10.7)	(6.46%–5.60%)	(3.1–10.7)
Black	11.76%	–9.36%	114.29%	23.15%	164.71%
	(1.7–1.9)	(2.99%–2.71%)	(2.1–4.5)	(4.19%–5.16%)	(1.7–4.5)
Hispanic	–30.00%	7.50%	52.63%	–20.52%	45.00%
	(2.0–1.4)	(4.00%–4.30%)	(1.9–2.9)	(6.87%–5.46%)	(2.0–2.9)
Age					
15–24	141.67%	N/A	75.00%	N/A	250.00%
	(1.2–2.9)		(2.4–4.2)		(1.2–4.2)
25–34	16.13%	N/A	143.75%	N/A	277.42%
	(3.1–3.6)		(4.8–11.7)		(3.1–11.7)
35–44	19.30%	N/A	67.90%	N/A	138.60%
	(5.7–6.8)		(8.1–13.6)		(5.7–13.6)
45–54	23.08%	N/A	91.36%	N/A	198.08%
	(5.2–6.4)		(8.1–15.5)		(5.2–15.5)
55+	23.08%	N/A	167.86%	N/A	240.91%
	(2.2–2.3)		(2.8–7.5)		(2.2–7.5)

Population					
1 million +	6.90%	24.93%	94.87%	–7.30%	162.07%
	(2.9–3.1)	(3.73%–4.66%)	(3.9–7.6)	(6.03%–5.59%)	(2.9–7.6)
Less than 1 million	36.00%	14.25%	109.52%	–19.50%	252.00%
	(2.5–3.4)	(4.28%–4.89%)	(4.2–8.8)	(6.82%–5.49%)	(2.5–8.8)
Not SMA or CMSA	52.38%	27.22%	129.73%	–33.08%	304.76%
	(2.1–3.2)	(3.60%–4.58%)	(3.7–8.5)	(5.29%–3.54%)	(2.1–8.5)
Total	18.52%	21.65%	102.50%	–11.26%	200.00%
	(2.7–3.2)	(3.88%–4.72%)	(4.0–8.1)	(6.13%–5.44%)	(2.7–8.1)

Source: CDC Wonder and 1999–2014 NSDUH.

The deadliness of prescription painkiller misuse, highlighted in Table 10, increased earlier and more rapidly than the deadliness of general prescription drug misuse. Between 1999 and 2001, the past-year prescription painkiller misuse rate increased by 27.9 percent, and prescription opioid overdose death rate increased by 35.7 percent. Past-year prescription painkiller misuse rates declined by 17.6 percent from 2002 to 2014, but prescription opioid accidental overdose rates more than doubled during the same period. In comparison, heroin use actually became less deadly from 1999 to 2001—past-year heroin use rates increased slightly during that period, while the heroin overdose death rate declined by 16.7 percent. As shown in Table 11, between 2002 and 2014 past-year heroin use rates more than doubled, but the heroin overdose death rate nearly quadrupled. All forms of prescription drug misuse have become much more deadly in recent years, but the increased deadliness of prescription painkiller misuse in the 2002–2014 period is particularly distressing. Similarly, the deadliness of heroin use increased at a pace that far exceeded the increase in the deadliness of any form of prescription drug misuse in this more recent period.

Demographic Trends in Prescription Drug Misuse Deaths

Like the demographic trends in prescription drug *misuse* rates described above, examining the demographic patterns in prescription drug misuse *death* rates are important for understanding why death rates have increased rapidly. Additionally, examining the trends in prescription drug misuse death rates among the various demographic groups will provide guidance for treatment and prevention strategies.

Gender

Males die from prescription drug misuse overdoses at a higher rate than females. As shown in Table 9, the prescription drug misuse overdose death rate was 8.2 per 100,000 males and 6.9 per 100,000 females in 2014. During the 15-year period between 1999 and 2014, however, the prescription drug misuse overdose death rate increased more rapidly for females than for males. Whereas the prescription drug overdose death rate more than doubled between 1999 and 2014 for males, the prescription drug overdose death rate for females more than tripled. The prescription drug overdose death rate also impacted females earlier; between 1999 and 2001, the prescription drug overdose death rate for males decreased by 12.1 percent but increased by 23.8 percent

Table 10. Prescription Painkiller Misuse and Opioid Overdose Death Rates, 1999–2014

	% Change Prescription Opioid Death Rate 1999–2001	% Change Past-Year Painkiller Misuse 1999–2001	% Change Prescription Opioid Death Rate 2002–2014	% Change Past-Year Painkiller Misuse 2002–2014	% Change Prescription Opioid Death Rate 1999–2014
Sex					
Male	25.00% (2.0–2.5)	27.68% (2.89%–3.78%)	112.12% (3.3–7.0)	–16.60% (5.06%–4.21%)	250.00% (2.0–7.0)
Female	55.56% (0.9–1.4)	25.00% (2.64%–3.30%)	157.89% (1.9–4.9)	–18.36% (4.14%–3.38%)	444.44% (0.9–4.9)
Race					
White	50.00% (1.6–2.4)	32.16% (2.83%–3.74%)	146.88% (3.2–7.9)	–19.53% (4.71%–3.79%)	393.75% (1.6–7.9)
Black	25.00% (0.8–1.0)	4.89% (2.25%–2.36%)	175.00% (1.2–3.3)	17.27% (3.59%–4.21%)	312.50% (0.8–3.3)
Hispanic	–33.33% (1.5–1.0)	9.51% (3.05%–3.34%)	53.85% (1.3–2.0)	–29.16% (5.35%–3.79%)	33.33% (1.5–2.0)
Age					
15–24	85.71% (0.7–1.3)	N/A	82.35% (1.7–3.1)	N/A	342.86% (0.7–3.1)
25–34	21.05% (1.9–2.3)	N/A	172.73% (3.3–9.0)	N/A	373.68% (1.9–9.0)
35–44	25.71% (3.5–4.4)	N/A	80.70% (5.7–10.3)	N/A	84.08% (3.5–10.3)
45–54	37.93% (2.9–4.0)	N/A	112.73% (5.5–11.7)	N/A	303.45% (2.9–11.7)
55+	33.33% (0.6–0.8)	N/A	354.55% (1.1–5.0)	N/A	733.33% (0.6–5.0)

(continued)

Table 10. *(continued)*

	% Change Prescription Opioid Death Rate 1999–2001	% Change Past-Year Painkiller Misuse 1999–2001	% Change Prescription Opioid Death Rate 2002–2014	% Change Past-Year Painkiller Misuse 2002–2014	% Change Prescription Opioid Death Rate 1999–2014
Population					
1 million +	12.50%	26.18%	116.00%	–17.76%	237.50%
	(1.6–1.8)	(2.75%–3.47%)	(2.5–5.4)	(4.56%–3.75%)	(1.6–5.4)
Less than 1 million	61.54%	24.50%	135.71%	–21.94%	407.69%
	(1.3–2.1)	(2.98%–3.71%)	(2.8–6.6)	(5.15%–4.02%)	(1.3–6.6)
Not SMA or CMSA	122.22%	38.37%	168.00%	–35.09%	644.44%
	(0.9–2.0)	(2.45%–3.39%)	(2.5–6.7)	(3.79%–2.46%)	(0.9–6.7)
Total	35.71%	27.90%	126.92%	–11.26%	321.43%
	(1.4–1.9)	(2.76%–3.53%)	(2.6–5.9)	(6.13%–5.44%)	(1.4–5.9)

Source: CDC Wonder and 1999–2014 NSDUH.

Table 11. Heroin Use Rates and Heroin Overdose Death Rates, 1999–2014

	% Change Heroin Death Rate 1999–2001	% Change Past-Year Heroin Use 1999–2001	% Change Heroin Death Rate 2002–2014	% Change Past-Year Heroin Use 2002–2014	% Change Heroin Death Rate 1999–2014
Sex					
Male	–16.67% (1.2–1.0)	66.67% (0.15%–0.25%)	333.33% (1.2–5.2)	96.15% (0.26%–0.51%)	333.33% (1.2–5.2)
Female	0.00% (0.2–0.2)	–6.25% (0.16%–0.15%)	650.00% (0.2–1.5)	155.56% (0.09%–0.23%)	650.00% (0.2–1.5)
Race					
White	–14.29% (0.7–0.6)	28.57% (0.14%–0.18%)	485.71% (0.7–4.1)	173.33% (0.15%–0.41%)	485.71% (0.7–4.1)
Black	12.50% (0.8–0.9)	220.00% (0.10%–0.32%)	177.78% (0.9–2.5)	3.03% (0.33%–0.34%)	212.50% (0.8–2.5)
Hispanic	–20.00% (1.0–0.8)	–27.78% (0.36%–0.26%)	111.11% (0.9–1.9)	50.00% (0.20%–0.30%)	90.00% (1.0–1.9)
Age					
15–24	0.00% (0.5–0.5)	N/A	450.00% (0.6–3.3)	N/A	560.00% (0.5–3.3)
25–34	0.00% (1.0–1.0)	N/A	627.27% (1.1–8.0)	N/A	700.00% (1.0–8.0)
35–44	–16.67% (1.8–1.5)	N/A	247.06% (1.7–5.9)	N/A	227.78% (1.8–5.9)
45–54	–7.69% (1.3–1.2)	N/A	235.71% (1.4–4.7)	N/A	261.54% (1.3–4.7)
55+	0.00% (0.1–0.1)	N/A	1300.00% (0.1–1.4)	N/A	1300.00% (0.1–1.4)

(continued)

Table 11. *(continued)*

	% Change Heroin Death Rate 1999–2001	% Change Past-Year Heroin Use 1999–2001	% Change Heroin Death Rate 2002–2014	% Change Past-Year Heroin Use 2002–2014	% Change Heroin Death Rate 1999–2014
Population					
1 million +	–11.11%	45.00%	290.00%	146.67%	333.33%
	(0.9–0.8)	(0.20%–0.29%)	(1.0–3.9)	(0.15%–0.37%)	(0.9–3.9)
Less than 1 million	–20.00%	–33.33%	440.00%	44.44%	440.00%
	(0.5–0.4)	(0.18%–0.12%)	(0.5–2.7)	(0.27%–0.39%)	(0.5–2.7)
Not SMA or CMSA	0.00%	250.00%	1300.00%	100.00%	1300.00%
	(0.1–0.1)	(0.04%–0.14%)	(0.1–1.4)	(0.06%–0.12%)	(0.1–1.4)
Total	–16.67%	25.00%	371.43%	117.65%	371.43%
	(0.7–0.6)	(0.16%–0.20%)	(0.7–3.3)	(0.17%–0.37%)	(0.7–3.3)

Source: CDC Wonder and 1999–2014 NSDUH.

for females. The faster growth in the prescription drug overdose death rate among females continued from 2002 to 2014. Although the overall prescription drug overdose death rate remained higher for males than females in 2014, the gender gap in the death rate narrowed substantially after 1999.

Importantly, prescription drug misuse became more deadly on a per yearly user basis between 1999 and 2014 for both males and females, and the more recent period between 2002 and 2014 showed a much more rapid increase in the deadliness of prescription drug misuse among females. Whereas the past-year prescription drug misuse rate decreased for females from 2002 to 2014, the prescription drug overdose death rate for females doubled over the same period. Males also experienced a decrease in the past-year prescription drug misuse rate from 2002 to 2014, but the prescription drug overdose death rate increased by 70.8 percent across this period for males. The deadliness of prescription drug misuse therefore increased substantially faster for females than males from 2002 to 2014.

As shown in Table 10, accidental overdose deaths from prescription opioid medications also increased substantially between 1999 and 2014 for both males and females, but the prescription opioid overdose death rate for females increased by a much larger percentage than for males during this period. Whereas the prescription opioid overdose death rate among males increased by 250 percent from 1999 to 2014, the same death rate for females increased by 444.4 percent. Even as the past-year prescription painkiller misuse rate decreased for both males and females from 2002 to 2014 by roughly equal percentages, the prescription opioid overdose death rate increased more substantially for females.

Trends in heroin overdose deaths shown in Table 11 also varied by gender between 1999 and 2014. The heroin overdose death rate was 5.2 per 100,000 males and 1.5 per 100,000 females in 2014. The heroin overdose death rate, however, increased much more rapidly for females than males between 1999 and 2014. By 2014, the heroin overdose death rate was 7.5 times higher than in 1999 for females and 4.3 times higher for males. Accounting for changes in past-year heroin use rates between 2002 and 2014 for males and females, the death rate per past-year heroin user more than tripled for males but quadrupled for females.

In sum, prescription drug overdoses are much more common among males than females, but the gender gap in prescription drug overdoses has decreased recently because of the more rapid increase in the prescription drug overdose rate among females between 1999 and 2014. Prescription opioid overdoses have become particularly problematic for females in recent years, and heroin overdoses, although much rarer than prescription opioid overdose deaths, are rapidly becoming a major crisis for females in the United States.

Race

Prescription drug misuse overdose deaths are higher for white Americans than for black and Hispanic Americans, as shown in Table 9. In 2014, 10.7 per 100,000 whites died because of an accidental prescription drug overdose, whereas 4.5 per 100,000 blacks and 2.9 per 100,000 Hispanics died of a prescription drug overdose in the same year. The race gap in prescription drug overdose deaths in 2014, however, was the result of a much more rapid increase in prescription drug overdose deaths among white Americans from 1999 to 2014 than among black and Hispanic Americans. Between 1999 and 2014, the prescription drug overdose death rate more than tripled for whites, nearly doubled for blacks, and increased by 45 percent for Hispanics. Because the past-year prescription drug misuse rate among white and Hispanic Americans decreased from 2002 to 2014 but the overdose death rates increased dramatically during this period, prescription drug misuse became much deadlier for these groups in recent years. Although the past-year prescription drug misuse rate among black Americans increased between 2002 and 2014, the overdose death rate increased at a much more rapid pace, showing that prescription drug misuse has become deadlier in recent years for black Americans too. The deadliness of prescription drug misuse, however, increased much more rapidly for white Americans than for black or Hispanic Americans during 2002–2015.

Similar patterns for prescription opioid overdose death rates are shown by race in Table 10, with the notable exception that black Americans experienced an increase in the prescription opioid overdose death rate closer to the percentage increase shown among white Americans than was shown for general prescription drug overdose death rates. The prescription opioid overdose death rate nearly quintupled for whites from 1999 to 2014, whereas the prescription opioid overdose death rate more than quadrupled for black Americans and increased by one-third for Hispanic Americans during this same period. Even with the dramatic increases in prescription opioid death rates for both black and white Americans during this period, white Americans continued to show a much higher prescription opioid overdose death rate (7.9 per 100,000) than black Americans (3.3 per 100,000) or Hispanic Americans (2 per 100,000) in 2014. Like overall prescription drug misuse overdoses described above, prescription opioid misuse has become much deadlier for all racial groups in the United States, but the deadliness of prescription opioid misuse has increased much more rapidly among white Americans.

As the prescription opioid overdose death rate increased very rapidly for white Americans from 1999 to 2014, the heroin overdose death rate shown in Table 11 among white Americans increased even more rapidly during this period. The heroin overdose death rate nearly quintupled for white Americans, more than tripled for black Americans, and nearly doubled for Hispanic Americans from 1999 to 2014. Like prescription drug overdose death rates described above, specifically in the form of prescription opioid overdose deaths, heroin overdoses are more common among white Americans (4.1 per 100,000) than black Americans (2.5 per 100,000) or Hispanic Americans (1.9 per 100,000) in 2014. Accounting for the past-year heroin use patterns by race, the deadliness of heroin use increased for all racial groups in the most recent period, 2002–2014, but unlike prescription drug misuse described above, the per yearly heroin user death rate increased more rapidly for black Americans than for white Americans or Hispanic Americans during this period.

Prescription drug misuse deaths have become primarily an issue among white Americans in recent years. Although prescription drug misuse rates generally and prescription opioid misuse specifically are not substantially more common among white Americans than black Americans or Hispanic Americans, the overdose death rates from prescription drug misuse are currently 2 to 4 times higher among white Americans. Heroin use rates are only slightly higher among white Americans, but the heroin overdose death rate is 1.5 to 2 times higher among whites than among black Americans or Hispanic Americans. Prescription drug overdose deaths as well as general opioid overdose deaths are therefore more heavily concentrated and are increasing more rapidly among white Americans.

Prescription drugs, especially prescription opiates, are killing an increasingly greater percentage of users from all races, but the increase in the deadliness of prescription medications has been much more significant for white Americans. In other words, the increase in prescription drug misuse rates does not explain the rapid increase in prescription drug overdose deaths—there is something about contemporary prescription drug misuse that is much deadlier now than in the past, especially for white Americans. Prescription drug misuse *deaths* among white Americans—mainly deaths caused by prescription opioid medications—is likely the reason for alarm among the public and policy makers. The connection between prescription opioid misuse/deaths and heroin use/deaths among white Americans is also likely a reason for public concern, which we investigate in detail in later chapters. Prescription drug and opioid misuse *deaths* might be the more important part of the racialization of the prescription drug misuse problem in the United States than prescription drug and opioid *misuse*.

Age

Because the age categories in the CDC Wonder system are different from the age categories in the NSDUH, no direct comparisons between prescription drug misuse and deaths by age can be made. That said, the age distribution of prescription drug overdose deaths can be tracked over time, and broad generalizations about the basic age distribution of use and deaths are possible. As shown in Table 9, prescription drug overdose deaths were primarily concentrated among Americans between 25 and 54 years of age in 2014. All age groups experienced rapid increases in prescription drug overdose death rates from 1999 to 2014, but the increases were slightly more rapid among those in the 15–34 and 55+ age ranges. Whereas the 35–44 and 45–54 age ranges experienced increases in the prescription drug overdose death rates of 138.6 percent and 198.1 percent, respectively, the younger and older age groups showed increases in prescription drug overdose death rates of 240.9–277.4 percent between 1999 and 2014. Prescription drug misuse deaths were more heavily concentrated among the middle-age groups in 2014, but the more rapid increases in prescription drug misuse deaths among the younger and older age groups in recent years have narrowed the age gap in prescription drug overdose death rates.

Not surprisingly, patterns of prescription opioid deaths from 1999 to 2014 shown in Table 10 were similar to patterns of overall prescription drug overdose deaths. Deaths from prescription opioid misuse are most common in the middle-age groups. In addition to the more rapid increase in prescription opioid overdose deaths than general prescription drug overdose deaths overall, the one notable difference in the patterns of deaths by age shown is that the oldest group experienced a much more significant increase for prescription opioid misuse deaths than general prescription drug overdose deaths from 1999 to 2014. The oldest group of Americans experienced a 733.3 percent increase in prescription opioid overdose deaths over the period 1999–2014. As evidenced in Table 11, even more stark increases in heroin deaths were shown for all age groups during this period, with the 55+ age group showing a 1,300 percent increase in heroin deaths from 1999 to 2014. Prescription drug misuse deaths are largely concentrated in the 18–34 age groups, but recent evidence shows that younger and older Americans have experienced very rapid increases in prescription drug overdose deaths in recent years.

Rural versus Urban

Although prescription drug misuse rates are generally lower in rural areas than urban areas, accidental death rates due to prescription drug overdoses shown in Table 9 are higher in rural areas than in major metropolitan areas. In 2014, 8.5 per 100,000 rural residents died from a prescription drug overdose, whereas 7.6 per 100,000 major metropolitan residents died of the same type of overdose. Residents in lesser populated metropolitan areas died of a prescription drug overdose at the rate of 8.8 per 100,000 residents in 2014. Both rural and urban areas experienced substantial increases in prescription drug overdose deaths from 1999 to 2014, but the largest increase in prescription drug overdose deaths was shown in rural locations. Prescription drug overdose death rates quadrupled in rural areas from 1999 to 2014, whereas prescription drug overdose death rates nearly tripled in major metropolitan areas and nearly quadrupled in smaller urban areas. Even though the past-year prescription drug misuse rate in rural areas decreased by 33.1 percent from 2002 to 2014, the prescription drug overdose rate increased by 129.7 percent during this period. Quite simply, deaths from prescription drug overdoses have become a much more significant issue in rural areas in recent years, even as the past-year prescription drug misuse rate in rural areas has dropped substantially. Accounting for changes in prescription drug misuse rates in rural areas, prescription drug misuse has become much more deadly per yearly user in rural areas in recent years.

Rural areas have a prescription drug misuse *death* problem, not a prescription drug *misuse* problem, in comparison with urban areas. Distressingly, prescription opioid misuse death rates shown in Table 10 increased even more rapidly from 1999 to 2014 in rural areas than in urban areas, with rural areas showing a 644.4 percent increase in the prescription opioid death rate during this period and major metropolitan areas showing a 237.5 percent increase in the prescription opioid death rate during the same period. Between 2002 and 2014, the past-year prescription painkiller misuse rate in rural areas decreased by 35.1 percent, but the prescription opioid overdose death rate increased by 168 percent during the same period. Heroin overdose deaths shown in Table 11 were nearly three times less common in rural areas than in major metropolitan areas, however, in 2014. That said, heroin overdose deaths increased by 1,300 percent in rural areas between 1999 and 2014. This increase in heroin overdose deaths mainly occurred between 2002 and 2014, when the past-year heroin use rate in rural areas doubled.

Drug use in any form is much less common in rural areas than urban areas, but overdose deaths have recently and increasingly become a major problem in rural areas. Deaths due to prescription drug overdoses generally and prescription opioid overdoses specifically have increased so substantially and rapidly in recent years that prescription drug overdose death rates in rural areas have superseded prescription drug overdose deaths in major metropolitan areas. Heroin overdose deaths are less common in rural areas than urban areas, but the rate of increase in heroin overdose deaths in rural areas recently has been extremely rapid. Stated simply, prescription drug overdose *deaths* are a major problem facing rural areas, but prescription drug misuse rates are much lower in rural areas than urban areas.

The New Face of American Drug Use

In this chapter, we have explored patterns of drug use and overdose deaths in the United States overall and among a variety of different demographic groups. The goals of this chapter were to show the extent of prescription drug misuse in the United States, understand the trends in prescription drug use over the past 20 years, determine if prescription drug misuse is concentrated among any specific demographic group, and investigate whether prescription drug misuse trends follow similar trends as other forms of drug use.

The main point to be taken from this chapter is that prescription drug misuse, in contrast to the depiction of the problem in media and political representations, is quite rare in the United States. Only 2.3 percent of Americans in 2014 reported abusing a prescription medication in the past month, and only 1.6 percent of Americans reported abusing a prescription painkiller in the past month. In 1994 prescription drug misuse was very rare, however, with approximately the same percentage of Americans reporting either prescription drug misuse or hard drug use. Prescription drug misuse certainly increased over the past 20 years, with prescription drug misuse being the second most commonly abused category of drug use in the United States in 2014, second only to marijuana use. Prescription drug misuse in 2014 was twice as common in the United States as hard drug use. Finally, although comparisons between the periods investigated in the current study are difficult due to methodological changes by the NSDUH, prescription drug misuse appears to have increased at a more rapid rate than either marijuana or hard drug use over the past 20 years. Although prescription drug misuse is relatively uncommon in the United States, there are plenty of reasons for the U.S.

population to be both hopeful and concerned about the prescription drug misuse problem.

There are many reasons for the U.S. population to be hopeful about the prescription drug misuse problem in the United States. For instance, there was a 10.1 percent decrease in past-month prescription drug misuse from 2002 to 2014, with the largest decrease in prescription drug misuse shown among the youngest Americans. Drug use patterns among youths and adolescents generally predict future drug patterns in the United States as a whole, so it is likely that the United States is nearing the end of the prescription drug misuse crisis that defined the late 1990s and early 2000s.

For every reason that Americans can be hopeful about the future of prescription drug misuse in the United States, however, there are just as many reasons for Americans to be concerned about the future of prescription drug misuse. The most significant concern is that the prescription drug misuse death rate has increased dramatically in recent years, even as prescription drug misuse rates have been declining. Prescription drug misuse is becoming more deadly in the United States, including among the youngest Americans. Even as fewer people in the United States are misusing prescription medications, a much greater number of Americans are dying from prescription drug overdoses. Perhaps the overwhelming attention on the prescription drug misuse problem in the United States by the media and politicians is less about the prevalence of prescription drug misuse in the United States and more about the consequences (i.e., death) of prescription drug misuse. The data presented in this chapter show that the United States does not have a prescription drug *misuse* problem; rather, the United States has a prescription drug overdose *death* problem.

The other major concern highlighted by the examination of drug use trends over the past 20 years is that as prescription drug misuse and prescription painkiller misuse have shown recent declines in prevalence in the United States, heroin use has increased. Although the prevalence of past-month heroin use is quite low in the United States, at less than 0.20 percent of the population in 2014, heroin use increased dramatically from 2002 to 2014 during a period in which prescription drug misuse decreased by 10.5 percent. It has been hypothesized that Americans are moving away prescription drug misuse and toward heroin use, and the data show that this a very possible trend. Later in this book, we explore the transition from prescription drug misuse and to heroin use, but for now it is important to point out that heroin use might be the next American drug trend. Heroin overdose deaths have also increased dramatically in recent years.

Prescription drug misuse represents a shift in the face of the American drug use scene. Prior drug use fads were portrayed as being an issue among young people, males, racial and ethnic minorities, the uneducated, urban residents, and the poor. To be sure, prescription drug misuse is currently more common among males than females, more common among black Americans than white Americans, more common among people below the age of 35 than older people, more common among high school dropouts than college-educated Americans, and more common in urban than rural areas. Taken at face value, prescription drug misuse patterns therefore look similar to patterns of other drug use trends. What makes prescription drug misuse unique, however, is that it is *relatively more common* among females, white Americans, older people, college-educated Americans, and rural areas than marijuana and some forms of hard drug use. In other words, prescription drug misuse has affected groups of Americans who have not traditionally been involved in other forms of drug use or drug use trends.

The story of prescription drug misuse is not about the percentage of people in the United States who misuse prescription drugs, however. Only 2.3 percent of Americans have misused a prescription medication in the past month, and this percentage has been decreasing in recent years among nearly every demographic group in the United States. Although there are many reasons to be concerned about the rate of prescription drug misuse in the United States, prescription drug *misuse* is not an epidemic in the United States. Rather, prescription drug misuse appears to have been a fad that emerged in the mid-1990s that lasted through the mid-2000s but has been subsiding in recent years.

The most concerning aspect of prescription drug misuse in the United States is the high and increasing rate of accidental prescription drug misuse overdose deaths. The rate of prescription drug misuse overdose deaths tripled from 1999 to 2014, and there is no evidence to suggest an end to the rapidly increasing prescription drug overdose problem. More people die of accidental prescription drug overdose each year than die of homicide or car accidents. If the United States in not experiencing a prescription drug *misuse* epidemic, it certainly appears to be is experiencing a prescription drug *death* epidemic.

Directly related to the public and political focus on the prescription drug misuse problem in the United States, the demographic trends in prescription drug overdose deaths show that the consequences of prescription drug misuse are affecting groups that were not traditionally involved in prior drug crises. Females, for instance, die of prescription drug overdose at a rate slightly lower rate than males, but the prescription drug overdose death rate increased almost twice as fast from 1999 to 2015 for females. Additionally, white Americans are more than twice as likely as black Americans to die of prescription drug overdose, and the rate of increase in the prescription drug overdose rate has been much faster among whites than blacks. Surprisingly, the 45–54 age group has the highest prescription drug overdose death rate of any age group, and older Americans have experienced rapid increases in prescription drug overdose death rates. Finally, the prescription drug overdose death rate in rural areas is now very close to or higher than the rate in urban areas, and rural areas have experienced the most rapid growth in prescription drug overdose death rates. In short, the groups that have been hardest hit by the consequences of prescription drug misuse are the groups that are least likely to be viewed as traditional drug users. Prescription drug misuse *deaths* are now primarily a problem among whites, older people, and rural areas and are quickly becoming a predominantly female problem.

Most important, the rate of prescription drug misuse overdose deaths has been increasing rapidly during a period in which prescription drug misuse rates in the United States have been decreasing. This means that a smaller percentage of the U.S. population is abusing prescription medications but that a higher percentage of Americans are dying from prescription drug overdoses. In other words, prescription drug misuse has become much deadlier on a per-user basis over the past 20 years.

The increased deadliness of prescription drug misuse is likely occurring for one of two reasons. The first explanation is that the shrinking number of prescription drug misusers in the United States are abusing prescription medications at a higher frequency and/or in higher doses. The second explanation is that the smaller percentage of prescription drug misusers in the United States are abusing prescription medications in more direct or dangerous ways (i.e., intravenously) or the prescription medications procured from street dealers are counterfeit and laced with more deadly substances (i.e., fentanyl). A full examination of the reasons for the increased deadliness are beyond the scope of this book, but prior researchers have shown statistically significant increases in the number of days on average that prescription opioids are misused in the United States from 2002–2003 to 2009–2010. The overdose death statistics reported by the CDC also show that fentanyl has become increasingly involved in prescription opioid overdose deaths. From 1999 to 2013, fentanyl accounted for less than 20 percent of all prescription opioid deaths, but 29 percent of prescription opioid overdoses in 2014 were caused by fentanyl. By 2015, 42 percent of prescription opioid deaths were caused by fentanyl.[4] It is possible that both an increasing frequency of prescription drug misuse among the declining number of prescription drug misusers *and* more dangerous forms of prescription drug misuse have coalesced to create the increasingly deadly prescription drug misuse problem. That said, prescription drug overdose deaths including prescription opioid overdose deaths have increased substantially in recent years even when fentanyl deaths are excluded. Fentanyl is part of the prescription drug misuse death problem but is far from the only factor in the increasingly deadliness of prescription drug misuse.

The reasons that prescription drug misuse has become more deadly notwithstanding, prescription drug overdose deaths cannot happen without a person first abusing a prescription medication. To more effectively combat prescription drug misuse, we must have a good understanding of the reasons that people misuse prescription drugs. The next chapter of the book therefore provides a comprehensive review of the causes of prescription drug misuse in the United States.

CHAPTER TWO

A Pill to Cure the Pain

In the previous chapter we described the facts of the prescription drug problem that has emerged in the United States over the past 20 years, a problem that is best evidenced by the dramatic increase in drug overdose deaths in recent years even as prescription drug misuse has decreased. The question remains, why do people misuse prescription medications? And if we understand some of the reasons, do they help explain the emergence, growth, and relative stability in prescription drug misuse?

In this chapter, we discuss why prescription drug misuse emerged as a popular from of drug use. We begin with a brief discussion of the history of drug use in the United States, as drug use has always been a part of our culture. Additionally, while drug users are often portrayed as outsiders or deviants, it is important to understand that millions of Americans are drug users. Findings from the 2016 National Survey on Drug Use and Health (NSDUH) indicate that 48.5 percent of Americans ages 12 and older—roughly 130 million people—have used an illegal drug at some point during their lifetime.[1] In order to fully understand prescription drug misuse in the United States, we also discuss the medical-industrial complex in this chapter. This term is used to describe the role played by the pharmaceutical industry, the medical profession (e.g., doctors and professional societies), and regulatory agencies. We specifically focus on the treatment of pain and how opioids came to be the go-to treatment for patients with chronic pain.

We also examine the academic literature on prescription drug misuse in this chapter. We begin with a review of the research on theoretical explanations for prescription drug misuse. Most of this research is within the field of criminology and focuses on the importance of social bonds, peer influence, exposure to strain or stress, and low self-control. We also revisit some of the correlates of prescription drug misuse discussed in previous chapters and attempt to provide some context for why females, whites, and rural residents are disproportionately more likely to misuse prescription drugs than engage in other forms of drug use. Additionally, we examine a factor that was not explored in the previous chapter—health insurance. Further, we address the motives for prescription drug misuse and patterns of diversion, or the various sources that people use to obtain prescription drugs. These concepts are important, because research shows that certain motives and sources of prescription drugs are associated with risky prescription drug misuse.[2] Finally, we tie it all together with a discussion of the prescription drug era that explains the role of broader cultural forces in the development, escalation, and cessation of prescription drug misuse in the United States.

Drugs in the United States

In the United States, the term "drug use" often brings to mind slogans such as "War on Drugs" and "Just Say No." Drug users are often viewed as being different and are stigmatized as being immoral or a threat to conventional society. Because of the negative view we have of drug users, our society uses the criminal justice system to regulate drug use. The current public health crisis created by prescription drugs has many people questioning this conventional wisdom. This is happening because many people who are suffering with prescription drug problems *do not fit the stereotypical view of drug users.* To better understand the shifting view of drug users from being in need of criminal justice intervention to being in need of drug treatment, it is important to understand that drug use has been a significant part of the U.S. culture for centuries.

American history, of course, begins with a discussion of indigenous Americans. We know that the use of naturally occurring plants or roots that had psychoactive properties was common among indigenous Americans.[3] For example, a small cactus that contains mescaline was commonly used for medicinal and religious purposes. Peyote has been consumed by indigenous Americans for centuries as part of religious ceremonies, not necessarily to get high. The belief that peyote could be used to cure physical and spiritual diseases led to peyote being incorporated into religious ceremonies as a holy sacrament. In part, peyote was used in religious settings for its hallucinogenic purposes. Consuming the drug frees the mind and allows one to make connections to the spiritual world. In addition, a side effect of peyote is that it often produces nausea and vomiting. This is an important part of the religious aspect of the drug's use, as vomiting was symbolically seen as a way to purge the body of both physical and psychological ills. While peyote is illegal in the United States today, an exception has been made for members of the Native American Church.

Alcohol is also a major part of U.S. society, as it is widely used and is a part of the regular lives of millions of Americans. Because of the widespread use of alcohol, Americans often do not think of alcohol as a drug, even though roughly 100,000 people die every year from alcohol-related issues.[4] Historians note that alcohol use has been part of the United States since the nation was settled by Europeans. Americans are familiar with the story of the Pilgrims, who settled in present-day Plymouth, Massachusetts, in 1620. Some historians believe, however, that the Pilgrims actually intended to settle in Jamestown, Virginia—a colony that was settled 13 years earlier—but had to shorten their trip because they ran out of beer. While this sounds far-fetched, it is well known that European settlers often brought alcohol with them when they crossed the Atlantic Ocean. During this age, people were unaware that microorganisms existed in water that at times made it unsafe to drink. The process of making beer involves boiling water, which killed off these microorganisms. In addition, beer was different 400 years ago and contained nutrients that helped supplement the diet of the time, and sailors believed that drinking beer prevented scurvy, a condition brought on by a lack of vitamin C that leads to a host of physical problems. Alcohol therefore has been a staple drug in the United States since its inception.

The way the U.S. government has viewed drug possession and use has changed dramatically over time. From the colonial era up to around the end of the 19th century, drug policy in the United States followed a laissez-fair approach. This is a French-derived term that is generally translated as "let them do what they want" and means that the U.S. government had very little regulation over how drugs were used medically or recreationally.

In colonial America, alcohol use was widely accepted. Beer, wine, and hard cider were often consumed during family meals and celebrations. Views of alcohol and other drugs in the United States, however, began to change drastically in the post–American Civil War era, leading to shifting policies on alcohol and other drugs in the late 19th and early 20th centuries. The sentiment to enact prohibition and criminalize alcohol, for instance, is often tied to the westward expansion of our nation, a period that marked a transition in the way Americans consumed alcohol away from the use of beer and wine in family settings to the use of hard liquor in saloons. Alcohol that was once consumed moderately in specific social settings became regular and heavy in public settings during the westward expansion in the United States. The saloon of the Wild West became associated with drunkenness, gambling, prostitution, and violence. Around this same time, the United States started to see an influx of immigrants who were "different" than the mainstream population. These immigrants were largely Catholic, not Protestant, and were from countries such as Italy and Ireland. As is still the case today, these immigrants were viewed as a threat to the existing American population with a different set of cultural values and as a source of economic competition. These immigrants often settled in the poorest urban neighborhoods that were marked by a variety of social problems, and alcohol was often identified as the problem when the real problem was oppressive social conditions such as economic inequality and discrimination.[5] The temperance movement developed shortly after the Civil War, and many states had already banned alcohol prior to the United States passing nationwide prohibition in 1920.

In addition to the changing public and legal perspectives on alcohol throughout U.S. history, drugs that are illegal today (e.g., heroin, cocaine, and marijuana) were all legal prior to the 20th century. These drugs were viewed like other commodities (e.g., corn, wheat, coal) that could be imported or exported on the global trade market. These drugs were also often ingredients in medicines or commercial products that were sold to consumers with little to no regulation. The most famous example may be Coca-Cola, which was invented in 1866 by Dr. John Stith Pemberton, a pharmacist in Atlanta, Georgia. Some 20 years earlier Pemberton mixed coca, a plant that contains the psychoactive alkaloid cocaine, and wine together. This style of drink was popular in France because of the euphoria caused from the mixture of alcohol and cocaine. As a pharmacist, Pemberton marketed his "French Wine Coca" as a general remedy for a wide variety of medical conditions. In 1886, however, Fulton County, Georgia, where Pemberton lived, enacted temperance legislation, making it illegal for him to sell his French Wine Coca. To be clear, his drink became illegal because the sale of alcohol, and not cocaine, was made illegal. At this point, Pemberton pivoted and added a sugar syrup in place of the wine, and the original formulation of Coca-Cola was born. Coca remained in the drink until 1903.

During this period, drugs such as opium and morphine were commonly used in everyday medications that were often given to children. Examples of this include Dover's Powder, which included opium, and Mrs. Winslow's Soothing Syrup, which included morphine. Introduced around 1850, Mrs. Winslow's Soothing Syrup was marketed to moms as a product that could soothe infants who were teething.

At the turn of the 20th century, drug policies in the United States began a dramatic shift. Three important laws were passed during this time. First, the Pure Food and Drug Act of 1906 required manufacturers to identify the ingredients in their products and restricted access to many drugs by making them available only via prescription. This law also created the Food and Drug Administration, a governmental regulatory agency that became responsible for the safety of over-the-counter and prescription medications. Second, the Harrison Narcotics Tax Act, passed in 1914, is one of the earliest antidrug laws passed in the United States. This law regulated and taxed the production, importation, and distribution of drugs such as heroin and cocaine. Finally, marijuana was effectively made illegal in 1935 with the passage of the Marijuana Tax Act.

The criminalization of drugs, however, did not bring an end to drug use in the United States. Since the end of World War II, nearly every decade has been marked by a major drug-related scare.[6] In the 1950s, it was heroin. Marijuana, amphetamines, and LSD dominated the 1960s. Quaaludes, barbiturates, and PCP were a major concern in the 1970s, and cocaine and crack dominated the 1980s. In the early 1990s methamphetamine reigned supreme, and prescription drugs came of age at the end of the decade. In the 2000s prescription drugs maintained their popularity, and novel psychoactive stimulants, such as synthetic marijuana and bath salts, became key players in the drug scene. For better or worse, drug use has been a part of American culture from the beginning.

Historically, research on drug use in the United States has focused on tobacco, alcohol, and so-called street drugs such as marijuana, cocaine, heroin, and methamphetamine. While prescription drugs have been around for decades, researchers did not carefully examine prescription drugs until the 1970s. For the sake of clarity, we use the general term "prescription drug misuse," throughout this chapter. Prescription drug misuse includes both medical misuse (the use of your own prescription medication in a manner that is inconsistent with doctor's instructions) and nonmedical misuse (the use of any prescription medication that has not been prescribed to you). Carl Chambers, the director of research for the New York State Narcotic Addiction Control Commission, pioneered prescription drug misuse research.[7] To understand the prevalence and correlates of prescription drug misuse, Chambers designed a general population survey that included questions related to prescription drug misuse and the diversion of prescription drugs. His efforts documented that prescription drug misuse was widespread in the 1970s and laid the groundwork for the inclusion of survey items related to prescription drugs to national epidemiological studies of substance use (e.g., the NSDUH, Monitoring the Future Study). The emergence of crack cocaine in the 1980s, however, pushed prescription drug misuse to the background in the world of drug research.

In the early 2000s, a report published by the National Center on Addiction and Substance Abuse at Columbia University shined a light on prescription drug misuse and propelled it to the forefront of substance use research.[8] Relying on several national epidemiological surveys of substance use, this report showed that prevalence rates of prescription drug misuse began to increase dramatically in the mid-1990s. While several different types of prescription drug misuse were reported, OxyContin misuse garnered the most media attention. In the late 1990s, OxyContin misuse began to take its toll in rural areas surrounding the Appalachian Mountains.[9] A number of factors contributed to this problem. First, many people living in these rural communities were employed in jobs related to manual labor, which produced many injuries or illnesses that resulted in chronic pain. Second, there was a lack of traditional drug distribution networks in rural areas. Drugs such as heroin and cocaine had historically been confined to urban areas. So, a population living with chronic pain and little access to traditional street drugs turned to OxyContin for self-treatment, cope with unfavorable rural living conditions, and get high.

This section outlined the history of drug use in the United States. Today, the United States is in the midst of a war on drugs whereby users are portrayed as being different from the rest of the population and a threat to our society's value system. It is important to remember, however, that drugs in a variety of forms have been a part of the American culture since before its inception, beginning with hallucinogens among indigenous Americans and alcohol in colonial America. The United States did little to regulate drugs until the 20th century, and drugs that are viewed as extremely dangerous today (e.g., heroin and cocaine) were once widely used in commercial products and over-the-counter medications. The antidrug movement in the United States began after the Civil War and focused on alcohol. In the last 100 years, several laws have been passed to regulate the use of drugs and send users to prison. This regulation, however, has done little to curb the use of drugs, as the United States has seen several drug epidemics in the last 60 years. We now turn our attention to a discussion of the reasons that prescription drug misuse became so popular in the United States over the past 20 years.

The Medical-Industrial Complex

In order to understand the current public health crisis associated with prescription drugs, it is important to look at the medical-industrial complex. This includes those employed in medical professions who have the ability to prescribe medications (e.g., physicians, physician assistants, nurse practitioners, dentists, and psychiatrists), pharmaceutical companies that develop prescription drugs, professional medical societies, and regulatory agencies.

One of the complications in understanding prescription drug misuse is that these drugs have legitimate medical uses. This is important because legitimate prescriptions are the primary source of prescription drugs for people who misuse prescription medications.[10] This includes people who misuse their own prescriptions, share their prescription drugs with friends and family members, and sell their prescription drugs to other people. Additionally, most people who develop substance use disorder symptoms related to prescription drugs initiated use via a legitimate prescription.

The medical use of prescription drugs is quite common in the United States. In 2016, 4.4 billion medical prescriptions were dispensed in the United States, up from 2.4 billion medical prescriptions in 1997. Prescription drugs are a big business in the United States, with more than $300 billion in sales reported in 2016. To fully understand the ubiquity of prescription drugs, data from the National Center on Health Statistics show that about 47 percent of adults in the United States report the medical use of at least one prescription drug in the past 30 days. Following trends in prescription practices is important, because the overprescription of drugs, primarily opioids, has been identified as a significant factor in the increase in prescription drug overdose deaths. While there are several classes of prescription drugs that are misused, including tranquilizers (e.g., Xanax, Ativan, Valium), stimulants (e.g., Adderall, Ritalin, Provigil), and sedatives (e.g., Ambien, Lunesta, Restoril), much of the public health problems are associated with the use of opioids (e.g., Vicodin, OxyContin, Tramadol). Opioids are prescribed primarily for the treatment of pain, so it is important to discuss pain from a medical perspective and how opioids became an acceptable treatment for people with chronic pain.

In her book *Drug Dealer, MD,* Dr. Anna Lembke examines the forces in addiction medicine that have contributed to the prescription drug crisis.[11] While Lembke focuses on the relationship between doctors and patients, she also discusses the role of pharmaceutical companies, professional societies, and regulatory agencies. Given that the current prescription drug crisis is largely driven by the use of prescription opioids, it is useful to begin with a discussion of the use of prescription opioids to treat pain. Historically, little attention was given to pain within the medical community. Pain was widely viewed as a symptom of an underlying condition and a part of the natural healing process of the human body.

Pain was therefore not viewed as a medical condition in need of treatment but rather as an acute problem that had an identifiable cause and lasted for a relatively short period of time. It was common for doctors to use medications to treat acute pain that was brought on by broken bones or surgery. Chronic pain, on the other hand, is more ambiguous for medical professionals. Chronic pain lasts for several months, and pinpointing the source or cause is often difficult. Historically, opioids were not used to treat chronic pain because there was a concern over their addictive nature. Pain management has become a major focus in health care today, as pain is now viewed as a problem to be avoided at all costs. Contemporary medicine now widely uses opioids to treat chronic pain. In fact, many doctors now view pain management as a moral obligation, and many medical professionals fear malpractice lawsuits if they do not effectively treat pain. Understanding the shift away from viewing pain as a symptom of an underlying medical condition to the use of opioids to treat chronic pain is essential for understanding how prescription drug misuse became more rampant in the late 1990s and early 2000s.

An important idea that dictates how doctors approach the treatment of pain today is compassionate care. This concept traces back to medical care provided to patients with a terminal disease. The basic idea was to allow patients with terminal illnesses to be as comfortable as possible. This in part explains the acceptable use of opioids among patients with terminal illnesses throughout U.S. history. There was less of a concern about negative outcomes such as addiction if a patient had a terminal condition or disease. The philosophy of compassionate care, if practiced more widely than for palliative care near the end of life, would mean the use of opioids for more medical conditions. After all, most people understand how simple day-to-day activities can become impossible when in pain, and many doctors have recently broadened the concept of compassionate care to the treatment of pain among patients who do not have a terminal illness.

The shift in the way doctors viewed pain and how it should be treated was heavily influenced by the pharmaceutical industry. In an effort to maximize profits, pharmaceutical companies have long attempted to influence how doctors treat their patients. Pharmaceutical companies traditionally attempted to influence medical professionals into prescribing their medications by providing information, sometimes misleading or inaccurate, about the effectiveness of their drugs. Pharmaceutical companies often fund research that highlights the effectiveness of their drugs that rely on small samples that are not generalizable to the broader population. During the 1980s, it was also a common practice for pharmaceutical companies to incentivize doctors to prescribe their medications. This practice generally involved providing gifts, meals, or travel to doctors and their family members but also occasionally involved direct payments. There are a number of examples of lawsuits filed against pharmaceutical companies over the last 30 years related to false claims regarding the safety or efficacy of their drugs. Many of these lawsuits ended in large financial settlements.

In an effort to enhance the credibility of their research, pharmaceutical companies began to provide funding to academic physicians in the 1980s who could be used as thought leaders to influence the medical field. During this period, a pro-opioid movement was fostered by the pharmaceutical industry with a goal of changing the way doctors thought about the treatment of pain. The goal was to have opioids become widely used to treat chronic pain among patients without terminal diseases. This was done by downplaying the risks associated with the long-term use of opioids, especially addiction, and convincing doctors that opioids were an effective and safe treatment for chronic pain.

Dr. Russell Portenoy was a well-known thought leader funded by the pharmaceutical industry who played an important role in how medical professionals viewed pain management. Portenoy, a pain specialist in New York City, published a highly influential article on the use of opioids to treat chronic pain.[12] His findings showed that opioids could be used to treat chronic pain on a long-term basis and that no dose of opioids was believed to be dangerous, and there was no evidence that opioids were addictive. While research such as this was promising, a single study should not be relied on to make major shifts in the treatment of pain. Portenoy's research did find evidence of compulsive use of opioids, a sign of addiction, but he claimed that compulsive use was due to the fact that his patients were in pain and needed their medication. Most problematic was that Portenoy's sample only consisted of 38 patients; it was not a random sample and the findings could not be generalized to a broader population. Also problematic was that the findings of his research were not empirically validated by other studies. Today much of Portenoy's research has been called into question, but during his time it had a dramatic impact on the medical field and how doctors thought about pain management.

In addition to these thought leaders, many pharmaceutical companies also created educational programs to shift the perception of prescription opioids. A major effect of these educational programs was to have pain recognized as a vital sign. In medical care, doctors gauge health and well-being with four vital signs (i.e., temperature, pulse, respiratory rate, and blood pressure). A major push occurred to have pain be adopted as the fifth vital sign. This was somewhat problematic, however, as objective indicators are normally used to measure vital signs. For example, a doctor can easily use a thermometer to determine if a patient is running a fever, indicative of a possible infection. However, there is no objective way to measure pain. Doctor's generally rely on a visual analog scale whereby patients report their subjective levels of pain on a numerical scale that often includes pictures of faces to show various level of pain. To date, there is little research showing that the use of these scales promotes better outcomes for patients—but the use of these scales does promote the use of opioids.

Much of the information included in these educational programs was funded by the pharmaceutical industry and used small nonrepresentative samples, and the findings were not empirically validated by additional research. These educational programs were used to target doctors, professional organizations (e.g., the American Pain Society), medical boards (e.g., the Federation of State Medical Boards), and accreditation organizations (e.g., the Joint Commission on Accreditation of Healthcare Organizations). From the outside these professional organizations appear to be legitimate, composed of academic researchers and medical professionals, but were often funded by the pharmaceutical industry and operated primarily as lobbying organizations. A key aspect of these organizations was the creation of guidelines for the treatment of chronic pain. Once the guidelines were established and adopted by a professional organization, the prescribing guidelines could be used to negatively label doctors who did not prescribe opioids to treat pain. These guidelines also opened doctors up to liability from malpractice lawsuits for medical professionals who did not prescribe opioids to treat pain. In addition, the guidelines made it difficult for state medical boards to regulate overprescribing by doctors. As long as a doctor was prescribing opioids to a patient to treat pain, in line with the guidelines established by the so-called professional organizations, there was little that could be done to control the prescribing practices of the doctor. The outcome of the thought leaders, educational programs, and professional organizations was to normalize prescribing opioids to treat pain, which placed tremendous pressure on doctors to prescribe opioids to patients who reported pain.

A few other important factors related to the prescribing practices of doctors that contributed to the growth of prescription drug misuse are worth mentioning. Quite interestingly, doctors receive little training on addiction in medical school or continuing education programs. Historically, substance abuse and dependence have not been core parts of the curriculum in medical school. This includes the field of psychiatry, which is surprising considering the overlap of mental health and substance use problems. Any training on addiction would come from a residency in addiction medicine or from their own experiences treating patients. The neglect of addiction training within the medical profession is likely due to how drug addiction has been widely viewed within American culture. Historically, drug use has been viewed as an individual choice, while addiction has been viewed as a sign of weakness or moral failing. This has begun to change, as addiction is now viewed as a chronic medical condition that requires treatment. The lack of training related to addiction, however, likely made it difficult for many doctors to identify the symptoms associated with drug abuse or dependence that their patients presented.

In addition, the doctor-patient relationship is built on mutual trust. It would be difficult for doctors to recognize that patients are lying to them about being in pain because they were simply seeking drugs to maintain an addiction. Related to this is the idea of illness narratives. With opioids being viewed as a safe way to treat chronic pain, the stigma associated with opioid use was removed. Drug addicts are highly stigmatized in the United States, viewed as weak moral failures prone to criminality and a threat to conventional values and beliefs. These illness narratives meant that people who became addicted to opioids were somehow different (i.e., better) than people who used heroin or other drugs. After all, people use heroin and other street drugs simply to get high, but people use prescription opioids to treat legitimate medical conditions. Ironically, it was the legitimization of opioids to treat pain that placed individuals with chronic pain at increased risk for addiction.

Another important aspect to discuss is access to health insurance. The treatment of addiction is quite expensive, a cost that many cannot afford if not covered in their health insurance plan. While health insurance policies will cover the prescription opioids that created the addiction, not all policies cover treatment for addiction. Some of this changed, however, with the passage of the Affordable Care Act (ACA), also known as Obamacare. Under the ACA, drug addiction was no longer considered a preexisting condition, and more insurance policies started to cover the expenses associated with treatment for addiction. Opioid treatment is also now available through the 1115 waiver for those Americans with Medicaid coverage in states that expanded Medicaid coverage under the ACA.

This section examined the medical-industrial complex and focused on how the medical profession viewed pain. Prior to the 1980s, pain was viewed primarily as a symptom of an illness and was only widely treated among patients with acute problems or those with a terminal illness. This chapter outlined the effort made to establish pain as a vital sign and showed how opioids came to be used to treat pain among those with chronic medical conditions. The pharmaceutical industry used thought leaders and launched educational programs to change the way people in the medical profession viewed pain and the use of opioids to treat pain, which laid the foundation for overprescribing medications and the development and expansion of prescription drug misuse. Similar efforts can be seen today with the direct-to-consumer marketing used by pharmaceutical companies. Pharmaceutical companies are now bypassing medical professionals and using commercials to inform regular people—potential customers—about diseases and medications that are used to treat those diseases.

Theoretical Explanations of Prescription Drug Misuse

The study of drug use is interdisciplinary, with academics from medical backgrounds, public health, psychiatry, psychology, social work, sociology, criminal justice, political science, and economics doing research in this area. Given that the use of a prescription drug that has not been prescribed to a person is against the law and that using prescription drugs in a manner inconsistent with a doctor's orders can be considered deviant, some social scientists view prescription drug misuse as a deviant/criminal behavior just like any other form of drug use. Criminology is one academic discipline that focuses its efforts on creating theory to understand crime and deviant behavior.

The primary frame of reference guiding contemporary criminological theory is positivism. Positivist criminology believes that behavior is largely shaped by factors that individuals cannot control, and criminologists seek to identify factors that place individuals at increased risk for crime and deviance. Some criminologists have a macro orientation and focus of structural characteristics that contribute to crime and deviance—for example, neighborhood characteristics. Other criminologists have a micro orientation and focus on important social process that contribute to crime and deviance—for example, the influence of family and peer interactions. To date, only a few criminological theories have been used to examine prescription drug misuse.

Social Disorganization Theory

Social disorganization is a macrolevel theory of crime that looks at community trends and patterns rather than individual differences in crime. In their study of rates of delinquency in urban areas, Clifford Shaw and Henry McKay found that certain neighborhoods had higher rates of delinquency than other neighborhoods.[13] Thus, social disorganization theory helps us understand how neighborhood characteristics influence deviance and crime. The theory focuses on factors such as high levels of poverty, physical decay, and broken families; rapid population growth; and an unstable heterogeneous population within neighborhoods. The resulting structural disadvantage has a devastating negative impact of social institutions (e.g., families and schools) and dramatically weakens the ability of a community to control the behaviors and activities within the neighborhood. More recent research on social disorganization examines how collective efficacy (the ability of neighbors to come together to solve common problems, build mutual trust, and regulate the behavior of others) and social capital (strong social ties between community members that create reasons to stay away from crime and deviance) link social disorganization to criminal behavior. These concepts recognize that strong ties between members of a socially disorganized neighborhood can work to prevent criminal activity.

To date, there is very little research using social disorganization theory to explain prescription drug misuse. One recently published study, however, used data from the National Household Survey on Drug Abuse and focused on adolescent respondents ages 12 to 17.[14] The research examined three different aspects of neighborhood characteristics: social disorganization (i.e., high rates of crime, abandoned buildings and graffiti, and a homeless population), social capital (i.e., neighbors help one another and often visit each other's homes), and social participation (i.e., involvement in peer mentoring programs, community centers, sports/clubs, volunteer or community work, and church activities). Findings indicated that adolescents who lived in neighborhoods with higher levels of social disorganization and with less access to social capital were more likely to report prescription drug misuse. These findings are consistent with the existing research on social disorganization and other types of drug use.

Social Learning Theory

The dominant perspective on social learning in the field of criminology is the theory put forth by Ronald Akers.[15] His social learning theory integrates the sociological concept of differential association,[16] which focuses on interactions with other people, with concepts from behavioral psychology,[17] which examines how behaviors are reinforced.

Social learning theory has four key concepts. First, focusing on interactions with other people, Akers uses the concept of differential association to highlight the importance of exposure to normative definitions. Interactions with other people who define substance use as acceptable increases the risk of substance use. These interactions, or associations, tend to have a more profound impact if they occur earlier in life (priority), more often (frequency), and for a longer period of time (duration) and are more salient to the individual (intensity). Second, the theory accounts for the modeling of other people's behavior with the concept of imitation. Akers argues that when people watch others participate in behaviors where they are rewarded, they are likely to model, or imitate, that behavior. Therefore, substance use is likely to be modeled if an individual witnesses others, particularly friends or family members, use drugs and experience positive outcomes. Third, to understand the attitudes and meanings that individuals attach to specific behaviors, Akers applied the concept of definitions. In particular, Akers noted that individuals would be exposed to a variety of definitions regarding behavior, so he focused on the balance of definitions that were either favorable or unfavorable to crime and deviance. When an individual possesses more favorable definitions, a behavior becomes more likely because these definitions frame the behavior as socially acceptable and make involvement advantageous. Finally, the concept of differential reinforcement focuses on the consequences that people attach to various behaviors. When positive consequences (rewards) outweigh negative consequences (punishments), that behavior becomes more likely in the future. In short, social learning theory argues that the causal mechanisms that explain deviant behavior involve interactions with primary group members (i.e., family and friends) who serve as deviant role models, provide normative definitions for crime and deviance, and reinforce deviant behavior.

A number of researchers have used social learning theory as a framework to understand prescription drug misuse among adolescents and young adults.[18] Supporting various elements of social learning theory, this research shows that prescription drug misuse is more common among individual who report prescription drug misuse among their close friends or peers. This finding is directly related to the concept of differential association, as drug use among friends/peers exposes one to others who define substance use as being acceptable. Drug use among friends and family members is also associated with imitation, as individuals may identify positive outcomes associated with drug use among their friends/peers. Finally, research also highlights the importance of attitudes toward substance use. Not surprisingly, when individuals think that drug use is more acceptable, they are more likely to report prescription drug misuse. This finding is consistent with the notion of definitions outlined in the theory. Interacting with friends or family members who define drug use also predicts prescription drug misuse, as prescription drug misuse is more common among respondents who report that friends and family members had more permissive attitudes toward substance use. Additional research testing the differential reinforcement component of social learning theory would provide a more detailed explanation of how other people can influence people to misuse prescription medications.

Control Theories

In general, control theories argue that people are naturally inclined to be deviant. Because of this view, control theories generally seek to explain why people conform to social norms and what mechanisms control deviant behavior. Hirschi's social bonding theory argues that people tend to conform when they internalize societal values and norms, or as Hirschi explained it, they developed a "bond" to society.[19] The social bond has four dimensions: attachment, commitment, involvement, and belief. Hirschi considered attachment to be important because it involved close affective ties to conventional others, such as parents or teachers. Strong attachment to others constrained deviant behavior, because involvement in such behavior would place these important social relationships at risk. Commitment focuses on the significance of investment in conventional activities and goals, such as education. Hirschi believed that commitment created a stake in conformity and that involvement in deviant behavior would be counter to this commitment toward a conventional life. Involvement is important because it consists of time spent in conventional activities, reduces time to engage in deviant behavior, exposes adolescents to conventional adults where attachments may develop, and involves participation in conventional activities, which all increase one's stake in conformity and therefore mitigate temptations to offend. Finally, belief is based on the internalization of societal rules and values. Individuals who believe in mainstream values avoid deviant behavior, because such behavior is counter to these mainstream values.

A number of studies have been published on social bonding and prescription drug misuse.[20] These studies tend to show that adolescents with weak bonds to either parents or school are at increased risk for prescription drug misuse. Given that research on prescription drug misuse shows that adolescents often obtain prescription drugs from their parents and misuse prescription drugs for conventional reasons (e.g., to get good grades), however, research on social bonds and prescription drug misuse must consider different types and motivations of prescription drug misuse. For instance, prescription drug misuse motivated by self-treatment might be more likely with stronger social bonds, whereas recreational misuse of prescription medication might be more likely with weaker social bonds.

Another control theory argues that behavior is constrained by self-control.[21] This general theory of crime argues that individuals who have low levels of self-control are more likely to engage in all types of deviant behavior. The theory focuses on inadequate socialization or poor parenting as a cause of low self-control. Individuals who have low self-control are thought to be impulsive, insensitive to the needs of others, physical as opposed to mental, risk takers, shortsighted, and nonverbal. Individuals with low self-control will have a difficult time resisting the immediate gratification associated with deviant behavior. This occurs because individuals with low self-control find it difficult to resist the immediate gratification that is associated with deviant behavior and fail to consider the long-term consequences that are associated with their actions.

Research also uses self-control to understand prescription drug misuse.[22] This research shows that key characteristics associated with low self-control (risk-taking and impulsivity) are associated with prescription drug misuse. Adolescents who like to take risks and are more impulsive are more likely to report prescription drug misuse. Again, research in this area must acknowledge that not all prescription drug misuse is the same. Aspects of low self-control may not be related to prescription drug misuse when the motive is self-treatment but could better explain prescription drug misuse when the motive is recreational.

Strain Theories

The concept of strain is based on the ideas of Émile Durkheim, one of the founding fathers of sociology. Durkheim proposed the idea of anomie to describe a state of normlessness, or a situation when the social norms used to control behavior break down. Simply stated, Durkheim believed that deviant behaviors were more likely when society was in a state of anomie. A number of criminologists have expanded on Durkheim's work and have applied the concept of anomie, or strain, to help explain deviant and criminal behavior. For the most part, strain theories argue that delinquency becomes more likely when it becomes difficult to achieve goals through conventional means. Rather than crime being inherent or natural for some people, strain theories argue that individuals are pressured into or resort to crime because they are unable to achieve important personal or cultural goals, such as monetary success.

Robert Agnew proposed a general strain theory that focused on micro-social interactions between individuals.[23] Agnew generally describes strain as being treated poorly by other people or as experiencing negative life events and outlined three primary sources of strain: failure to achieve positively valued goals (e.g., financial success or good grades in school), removal of a positively valued stimuli (e.g., loss of a job or end of a relationship), and the presence of noxious stimuli (e.g., being the victim of bullying or a crime). Agnew argued that strain increased the likelihood of crime, because strain resulted in a range of negative emotions such as anger, frustration, jealousy, depression, and fear. Deviant behavior is simply one possible way an individual can alleviate strain or the negative emotions that accompany strain.

Much of the research involving strain and prescription drug misuse involves general strain theory and identifying different types of strains that are related to prescription drug misuse.[24] Research shows that experiencing negative life events (e.g., fights with parents, bad grades in school, not living with both biological parents, not having health insurance, poverty, and poor overall health) is associated with prescription drug misuse. Some research examines specific types of strain (e.g., bad grades, work-related stress, and poor health) and prescription drug misuse. This research shows that strain is associated with prescription drug misuse because strain is associated with depression or other forms of psychological distress. Given the conceptual overlap between what sociologists label as strain and how public health researchers describe stress, general strain theory offers a very useful framework for the study of prescription drug misuse that is related to both self-treatment and recreational motives.

Life-Course Theories

The life course has become a dominant perspective in the field of criminology. While traditional theories of crime and deviance, such as those that have been reviewed so far, tend to focus on the initiation of criminal acts among adolescents, focus on the life course examines a multitude of factors that shape offending behavior from adolescence to adulthood. Life-course theories tend to examine developmental trajectories over time, including the factors that cause deviance/criminal behavior during the transition from adolescence to adulthood.

The life-course theory approach argues that events that occur in adolescence are causally related to events that happen later on in life. The theory contends that a process of cumulative disadvantage creates stability in offending behavior over time, as involvement in deviance/crime at an early age tends to limit future opportunities and options for a conventional life, especially when an individual is arrested. Life-course theory also examines transitions that can redirect developmental trajectories toward or away from crime and deviance. While most adult criminals began breaking the law when they were adolescents, most adolescents who break the law stop doing so when they become adults. Life-course theory seeks to identify important transitions that create turning points and lead to desistance, such as getting married or finding a good job in adulthood.

The leading proponents of the life-course approach in criminology are Robert Sampson and John Laub, and their theory of age-graded informal social control has been guided by two principles.[25] First, antisocial behavior in adolescence is linked to criminal offending during adulthood through the process of cumulative disadvantage, or the process by which early criminal offending mortgages the future by limiting future engagement with conventional others and institutions. Second, salient life events and social ties embedded in adult transitions explain variations in criminal offending that are unaccounted for by childhood predictors. The significance of the life-course approach lies in the study of desistence, or the process of the discontinuation of criminal activity.

Limited research applies the life-course theory to prescription drug misuse. A few notable studies, however, look at the link between life events and prescription drug misuse among adults or desistence from prescription drug misuse. A study by Gunter et al. examined patterns of desistance from prescription opioid misuse to see if it was similar to illicit drug use.[26] The data they used came from the South Beach Project, a sample of 600 ethnically distinct polydrug users in Miami-Dade County, Florida. The results found that an association with antisocial or drug-using peers hindered the desistence process for nonmedical prescription opioid users. This supports a life-course perspective that emphasizes the significance of social bonds in desistence from drug use. Dollar and colleagues published two studies that examine the relationship between adult social bonds and prescription drug misuse.[27] This research found that marital bonds and work satisfaction were inversely related to prescription drug misuse, meaning that people with strong marriages and stable work were less likely to misuse prescription medications. In addition, respondents who were employed were less likely to report prescription opioid misuse. The life-course framework is an important theoretical perspective, as it can be used to understand both stability and change in prescription drug misuse over time. To understand why use continues over time, the theory focuses on the cumulative disadvantage of early prescription drug misuse and the weakening of social bonds that occurs as the result of prescription drug misuse. To explain changes in drug use over time, the theory highlights the development of strong social bonds in adulthood that lead prescription drug misusers to stop abusing prescription medications.

Additional Theoretical Perspectives

Research outside of sociology/criminology has also offered theoretical explanations of prescription drug misuse. A few researchers have relied on the theory of planned behavior, which is commonly used to understand health-related behaviors.[28] Grounded in the theory of rational choice, the theory of planned behavior contends that individuals weigh rewards and consequences prior to engaging in a behavior. To understand how these decisions are made, or more precisely the intentions that people have to engage in a behavior, the theory focuses on attitudes, subjective norms, and perceived behavioral control. Research in this area is generally supportive of the theory of planned behavior in predicting prescription drug misuse among adolescents and young adults.[29] Most of the research in this area relies on samples of college students, looks at the misuse of prescription stimulants, and highlights the importance of subjective norms and attitudes about prescription drug misuse.

Other researchers have relied on the theory of triadic influence, an ecological model, to study prescription drug misuse.[30] Much like the theory of planned behavior, the theory of triadic influence seeks to explain health-related behaviors. It can be viewed as an integrated theory that combines many concepts from the theories we have already discussed. The theory identifies different streams of influence (e.g., intrapersonal, social context, and sociocultural environment) and various levels of causation (e.g., ultimate, distal, proximal, and immediate precursor). The small amount of research on prescription drug misuse has provided empirical validation for many aspects of the theory.[31]

This section reviewed the existing research that has offered theoretical explanations for prescription drug misuse. The majority of this research relies on several empirically validated theories from the field of criminology. This research focuses on the importance of strong social bonds (e.g., family, school, and employment), the importance of attitudes and behaviors of others (primarily peers), the impact of experiencing strain, and low self-control. In addition, one study focused on neighborhood characteristics and showed that prescription drug misuse is more likely in neighborhoods that are socially disorganized. To develop effective prevention and interventions related to prescription drug misuse, continued research on theoretical explanations is needed. In particular, research identifying how prescription drug misuse is different from other types of drug use would be particularly useful.

Correlates of Prescription Drug Misuse

In the previous chapter, we reviewed demographic patterns associated with prescription drug misuse and identified that prescription drug misuse was disproportionately more common than other forms of drug use among some groups that are generally not viewed as drug users, including females (vs. males), whites (vs. blacks), and rural residents (vs. urban residents).

Gender

With regard to gender, males generally have higher rates of involvement in criminal behavior and substance use than females. However, an interesting finding has emerged in the prescription drug misuse literature. A number of studies using nationally representative data have found that adolescent females between 12 and 17 years old are at increased risk for prescription drug misuse compared to males of the same age range. It should be noted that this relationship tends to flip with age, as among adult populations, gender is sometimes not significant or males are at increased risk for prescription drug misuse. There is little research that examines gender and prescription drug misuse, and the growing problem of prescription drug misuse among adolescent females clearly needs to be a focus of future research.

One possible explanation for increased risk of prescription drug misuse among females is likely how prescription drugs are viewed in U.S. culture. First, there is a perception that prescription drugs are not drugs, at least not in the same sense that cocaine and heroin are viewed as drugs. Thus, there is less social stigma associated with the misuse of prescription drugs. Second, prescription drugs are much more widely available than traditional street drugs, and the sources of prescription drugs are less risky and stigmatizing. The most common sources of prescription drugs are friends and family members or a prescription from a doctor. Not having to obtain drugs from a dealer therefore might be an important factor driving prescription drug misuse among females. Prescription drugs are also viewed as being safer than traditional street drugs, as people believe that there is less chance of negative consequences, both physical and social, associated with prescription drug misuse. The lower perceived social and health risks associated with obtaining and misusing prescription medications, compared with other drugs, is likely a key factor that explains the greater involvement of females in prescription drug misuse.

General strain theory also offers some evidence for why females are overrepresented in prescription drug misuse patterns.[32] Research using general strain theory suggests that strain is a gendered process in that men and women are exposed to different types of strain, and men and women also respond to strain in different ways. One important gender difference is that women tend to respond to strain with depression rather than anger. This is important, because depression is strongly associated with prescription drug misuse, whereas anger is a more likely reaction to strain for males and is associated with overt physical actions such as violence. Gender differences in prescription drug misuse therefore can be explained by a combination of risk assessments and gender socialization practices, but additional research is needed to better identify the reasons that females are disproportionately likely to misuse prescription medications.

Race

The statistics outlined in the previous chapter show that whites are also disproportionately likely to report prescription drug misuse than are racial and ethnic minorities in the United States compared with the use of most other drugs. There is a general stereotype in American society that drug users are largely minorities, but that view is not supported by the prescription drug misuse statistics. Some substance use research suggests that a race-age crossover effect exists.[33] This research shows that among adolescents and young adults, whites tend to have the highest prevalence rates of most types of substance use. This relationship, however, changes around age 35, the age at which statistics start to show that substance use is more prevalent among blacks than among whites. This pattern is particularly strong for black males, who are more likely than any other combination of race and gender to report drug use later in life. The trends described in the previous chapter suggest that the race/ethnic age crossover effect is evident for prescription drug misuse, as prescription drug misuse among black Americans continued to increase in the most recent period examined, even as prescription drug misuse among white Americans declined, and that prescription drug misuse is more "sticky" among blacks than whites.

There are also some risk factors for prescription drug misuse that are related to race/ethnicity.[34] To date, only a small body of research has examined the difference in risk factors for prescription drug misuse by race and ethnicity, and what limited research exists finds that risk factors for drug use tend to be similar across race/ethnicity. Research on prescription opioids, however, specifically shows that gender is a significant predictor for prescription opioid misuse for blacks but not whites. That is, black males are at increased risk for prescription opioid misuse than are any other combinations of race and gender. In addition, being on a government program is also a significant predictor of prescription opioid misuse for blacks but not whites.

The statistics outlined in the previous chapter highlight that prescription opioid misuse has become more common among blacks. Research has shown that there are some unique risk factors for substance use in general among black Americans. The most important risk factors for drug use are perceived discrimination, structural disadvantage, and subcultural norms. Scholars such as John M. Wallace Jr. have emphasized *racialized social systems* to understand substance use among blacks in the United States, focusing mainly on adverse social conditions related to lower social status.[35] These adverse conditions, however, can sometimes work as protective factors. For example, black adolescents are more likely to experience and witness the negative consequences associated with substance use. Black adolescents often have a firsthand view of the impact that drugs have on their family members, friends, and community as a whole. This process explains why children growing up in the 1980s who saw the negative experiences with crack turned to marijuana use, specifically blunts, when they reached adolescence and young adulthood in the 1990s. These negative consequences may also make black parents protective of their children and keep them away from dangerous drugs. To explain the race-age crossover effect, it is important to look at how social factors change over time. Research shows that blacks are less likely to get married than whites, which is important given that married adults, particularly males, have lower rates of substance use and prescription drug misuse. In addition, some research suggests that the effects of poverty become more pronounced over time—as blacks age, the thought of achieving the American Dream becomes less realistic, which might lead to an attitude marked by alienation and hopelessness, both of which are strong predictors of prescription drug misuse.

Geographic Residence

There is considerable evidence that prescription drug misuse, particularly opioids, began as a rural problem. As explained earlier, parts of

Appalachia had large numbers of people who had chronic medical conditions that produced pain. Today, prescription drug misuse is not a strictly rural problem. Although prescription drug misuse prevalence rates were higher initially in rural areas, there are little differences in prescription drug misuse prevalence rates today between rural and urban locations. However, heroin is noticeably an urban drug, as heroin has not yet infiltrated rural areas. There is simply greater access to prescription drugs in rural areas compared to traditional street drugs such as heroin and cocaine that are generally distributed in open-air drug markets in impoverished urban neighborhoods. Research therefore needs to look at geographic residence and understand the similarities and differences in prescription drug misuse in urban, suburban, and rural places.

Researchers such as Katherine M. Keyes have identified a number of factors to consider when examining geographical differences in prescription drug misuse.[36] First, it is important to focus on macrocharacteristics such as access to drugs. As we established earlier, a large portion of the country uses drugs, and the particular drug they use may be based simply on availability. Second, normative perceptions associated with drug use are also important to consider in both rural and urban locations. As we have discussed, there is a perception that prescription drugs are safer than street drugs and that many people misuse prescription drugs for conventional reasons, not to get high. It is important to examine how these normative perceptions vary by geographic residence and how these attitudes may account for drug use outside of urban areas. This is important, because drug use has stereotypically been viewed as an urban problem in the United States. Finally, it is also important to identify how sources of structural stress (e.g., discrimination and economic inequality) vary by geographic residence.

A few aspects of life in rural areas are also important to discuss. First, adults who live in rural areas may be affected by a greater number of risk factors for prescription drug misuse. The negative impact of economic conditions in rural areas is especially important, as many young adults will migrate from these areas to pursue better economic opportunities, leaving the adults who remain in rural areas to experience greater economic stress and loneliness, both of which might increase the risk for prescription drug misuse. When focusing on adolescents in rural and urban areas, it is important to identify possible differences in family and peer influence by geographic location. Research suggests that social networks are denser in rural areas and tend to be centered on family and work relationships. Given that we know that family members and friends are a common source of prescription drugs, it is important to examine how these social networks influence substance use in rural areas.

Health Insurance and Unemployment

An interesting finding from the research on prescription drug misuse has emerged and is in need of further exploration. A number of studies show a correlation between health insurance status and prescription drug misuse—respondents with no health insurance are at increased risk for prescription drug misuse.[37] It is important to determine the causal mechanisms that link health insurance and prescription drug misuse. The motivations for prescription drug misuse are possibly associated with health insurance status, as individuals who do not have health insurance might be more likely to misuse prescription drugs to self-treat. Without health insurance, access to health care is limited, so a person with no insurance who is dealing with chronic pain may be forced to turn to family or friends to provide them with prescription opioids, as they are unable to obtain these medications from a doctor. On the other hand, the relationship between health insurance status and prescription drug misuse may be more complex. It is important to understand the unique risk factors that people without health insurance face. Perhaps the differences between people with and without health insurance account for the relationship between health insurance and prescription drug misuse. As health insurance is often tied to employment, it is important to note that the unemployed consistently have higher rates of substance use, including prescription drug misuse, than those who work part- or full-time.[38] The role of health insurance therefore might directly influence prescription drug misuse through the process of self-treatment or might indirectly contribute to the prescription drug misuse problem through spurious characteristics that predict both not having health insurance and engaging in prescription drug misuse, including employment status.

Motives and Sources of Diversion

Motivations

There is a good amount of research on the motivations for prescription drug misuse, but much of the early research on motivations relied on samples of students and was not generalizable to the population of the United States. To address this problem, the NSDUH redesigned the module of survey items associated with prescription drugs. One significant addition was questions on motivations for specific categories of prescription drugs (e.g., opioids, tranquilizers, stimulants, and sedatives).[39] Motivations generally fall into two categories—self-treatment and recreational.

Data from the 2015 NSDUH shows that the most common motives are related to self-treatment. For prescription opioids, the most common motive was to relieve physical pain (63 percent). The two most commonly mentioned motivations for prescription tranquilizer misuse were to relax/relieve tension (45 percent) and help with sleep (21 percent). For prescription stimulants, the most common motivations were to help be alert or stay awake (27 percent), help concentrate (27 percent), and help study (23 percent). Finally, for prescription sedatives by far, the most common motivation listed was help with sleep (72 percent). To assess recreational motives, the NSDUH specifically asks respondents if they misused prescription drugs "to feel good or get high." Roughly 12 percent of respondents mentioned recreational motives for opioids, 12 percent for tranquilizers, 11 percent stimulants, and 6 percent for sedatives. The data clearly show that self-treatment is the primary factor behind prescription drug misuse.

It is important to assess motivations for prescription drug misuse to help understand risk associated with misuse. For example, taking a stimulant without a prescription to study for an exam is a different type of drug use than taking a prescription opioid to get high. In fact, some research highlights the importance of motivations by showing that recreational motives are more strongly related to more frequent misuse of prescription medications, substance use disorder symptoms associated with prescription drugs, and the use of other illicit drugs.[40] Prescription drug misuse comes in many different forms and is motivated by many different factors, but the form and motivation for prescription drug misuse is critically important for understanding the degree, scope, and consequences of prescription drug misuse.

Diversion and Sources of Prescription Drugs

Generally, diversion is defined as the transfer of controlled drugs from a lawful to an unlawful channel of distribution. There is little reliable data on patterns and trends in the diversion of prescription drugs over time. One source of data, which is not publicly available, is the Researched Abuse, Diversion and Addiction-Related Surveillance (RADARS) system. RADARS collects data from several sources including poison control centers, medication-assisted treatment programs, patients entering treatment for substance dependence, drug diversion and regulatory agencies, and general population samples. To estimate prescription drug diversion, RADARS collects data from law enforcement agencies, pharmaceutical boards, and departments of health. Data from RADARS show large increases in the diversion of prescription opioids from 2002 to 2010, with rates stabilizing or even slightly decreasing from 2011 to 2013.

Because diversion is difficult to measure in empirical research, diversion is defined in most surveys as how people obtain the prescription medications that they misuse. The NSDUH has asked respondents about sources of prescription drugs for years.[41] Sources of prescription drugs are generally broken into three distinct groups: health care provider, friend or relative, and bought from a dealer or a stranger. The health care provider source includes from one doctor, from more than one doctor, or stolen from a doctor's office, clinic, hospital, or pharmacy. The friend or relative source includes from a friend/relative for free, bought from a friend/relative, or stolen from a friend/relative. The NSDUH assesses sources of prescription drugs from separate categories of prescription drugs. The following findings are from the 2015 NSDUH and highlight the most common sources of prescription drugs mentioned by respondents. For all prescription drugs, the most common source was from a friend or a relative for free (opioids, 41 percent; tranquilizers, 51 percent; stimulants, 56 percent; and sedatives, 57 percent). The second most common source was from one doctor (opioids, 34 percent; tranquilizers, 21 percent; and sedatives, 27 percent). The third most common source among stimulants was bought from a friend or family member (20 percent). Interestingly, a small proportion of respondents reported bought from a dealer or a stranger as a source (opioids, 5 percent; tranquilizers, 8 percent; stimulants, 5 percent; and sedatives, 3 percent). Clearly, friends and family are the primary way that people obtain the prescription medications they misuse.

Identifying sources of prescription drugs is important for several reasons. First, source is associated with patterns of prescription drug misuse. Research shows that certain sources (i.e., bought from a dealer or stranger) are more strongly associated with more frequent misuse of prescription drugs, substance use disorder symptoms associated with prescription drugs, and the use of other illicit drugs than other sources (i.e., from a friend or family member for free).[42] Research on sources is also important to help develop effective prevention and intervention strategies. The most common sources are parents and doctors. Parents need to understand the risks associated with prescription drugs and not provide their children with those substances. Likewise, doctors need to understand that some of their patients are addicted.

Research on motives and sources of diversion are important in that they help contextualize prescription drug misuse. For example, it is pretty clear that the use of opioids to get high is not the same as the use of simulants to help study. Likewise, using prescription drugs that were given to you by a friend or family member for free is different than buying prescription drugs from a drug dealer. The existing research in this area clearly shows that certain motives and sources are associated with risky drug use (e.g., more frequent use, substance use disorder symptoms, and the use of alcohol and other drugs). This research highlights that not all drug use and users are the same. Some people use drugs for conventional reasons (e.g., to self-treat or study), some acquire drugs from conventional sources, and some patterns of drug use increase the risk for negative outcomes. What is clear, however, is that the small percentage of people who obtain prescription medications to misuse for recreational purposes through drug dealers are at the greatest risk for frequent misuse and the negative consequences (i.e., death) of prescription drug misuse.

Drug Generations

A theory of subcultural evolution advanced by Golub and his colleagues may help us understand how we got to where we are today.[43] Based on extensive research on drug users, this theory focuses on culture and identity development to understand how the popularity of certain drugs shifts over time. Culture is of particular importance, because it establishes both a moral and a behavioral imperative for drug use patterns. That is, culture teaches us how to think about what is happening around us and how to act in certain situations. Culture also helps us to understand the symbolic meaning that individuals attach to drug use. That is, why do individuals use drugs, and what does their drug use mean to them? To understand this, one must understand drug subcultures.

A subculture is generally viewed as a culture within a culture, or a group that shares many of the same values and norms as society as a whole but embraces a few values and norms that set them apart from the dominant culture. An examination of subcultures helps us understand how the symbolic meaning attached to specific drugs changes over time and how the current drug of choice is defined as normative within the subculture. The theory is important in that it outlines how the subculture shapes the way certain drugs are viewed, including what drugs are acceptable and available to use, the symbolic meaning attached to a specific drug, how use determines affiliation within a subculture, and the consequences associated with use or nonuse. While conventional wisdom casts drug use as an individual decision, this theory argues that drug use patterns cannot be understood without examining the values and norms of subcultures and how drug use is associated with identity and affiliation in certain social groups.

Golub et al.'s theory also stresses the importance of identity, how drug use is used as a way for individuals to establish their identity and find friends. Sociologists generally focus on social interactions with others to understand how one's self-concept develops over time. These interactions shape one's self-concept by helping them understand which attitudes and behaviors are accepted by various groups. If someone wants to be a part of a group, he or she will adhere to the norms and the values of the group. Think of an adolescent who aspires to be a professional athlete—the individual understands that the norms and values associated with being an athlete involve dedication, sacrifice, and hard work. To be accepted as an athlete by one's teammates and coaches, adherence to those norms and values is essential. So, adolescents who are interested in drug use look to these existing subcultures (made up of family members, peers, or members of the community) to understand the norms and values of the group they want to be a member of. These adolescents learn which drugs are popular, why and how people use drugs, and how drug use facilitates access to the subculture.

This theory has been used to describe what Golub and colleagues call drug eras and understand the social factors that influence the popularity of specific drugs over time.[44] The term "era" is specifically used instead of the term "epidemic" due to the pejorative nature of the word "epidemic," which creates a stigma associated with use. Building on Zinberg's classic research on set and setting, Golub and colleagues focus on the social and cultural influences associated with drug use.[45] To frame drug eras, they identify four distinct phases. First, incubation involves a specific drug being used by a relatively small segment of the population, generally within a specific social context. Symbolic meaning is important here, as users at this stage get in on the ground floor, if you will. It is like someone saying that he or she liked a rock band before the band became popular. Second, expansion occurs when the drug becomes more available and more people begin to use. Individuals who initiate drug use during the incubation phase are generally of high social status within drug subcultures. Drug use shifts to the expansion phase when people who aspire to be of higher social status within their peer groups gain access to the drug. This goes back to the symbolic meaning of drug use and how individuals will use drugs to shape their identity and facilitate membership to specific subcultural groups. The third stage, or plateau, involves widespread use of the drug. It occurs when basically everyone with an interest in drug use and also has access to the drug has used it. This is when the drug becomes the most popular drug, and all adolescents who come of age will seek out this drug. Symbolic meaning is also important at this phase, as most social activities and relationships within certain groups will revolve around this drug. Finally comes the decline phase. A drug declines in popularity for several reasons, but this theory focuses on normative expectations associated with a specific drug. Normative expectations of a specific drug will likely change when negative consequences associated with the drug become widespread, including criminal sanctions, general social stigma, or health-related problems. Also, a drug may simply lose its luster; after being around for a while, it may no longer be perceived as the cool drug and will likely be replaced by a new drug. During this decline phase, the prevalence of use will decline among the population as a whole, but many are likely to continue use as a means to support an addiction that has developed over time.

This theory places a special emphasis on adolescents and young adults, specifically those who come of age during a particular drug era. The initiation of drugs is common among adolescents and young adults. Without firsthand experience with drug use, adolescents and young adults will often seek out whatever drug is most popular or readily available. Adolescents and young adults are also susceptible to the normative expectations of others as they seek to create an identity and belonging in certain social groups.

The Prescription Drug Era

Golub and his colleagues have used this theory to identify previous drug generations, including a heroin generation, a crack generation, and a blunt generation.[46] Relying on the core principles of this theory, we outline the cultural norms that helped bring prescription drugs, primarily opioids, to the forefront of the drug world. It is important to remember that alcohol and other drug use is very much a part of American culture and has been for centuries. So, the use of drugs should not be a surprise, but this theory relies on drug subcultures and people's social position relative to these subcultures to understand why certain drugs become popular. These issues are important, because they impact which drugs are acceptable and available to use, the symbolic meaning attached to drug use, how drug use is related to identity and group affiliation, and the consequences of drug use.

An important idea to discuss is the perception of prescription drugs compared to traditional street drugs. Importantly, the use of prescription drugs is perceived to be more socially acceptable. This is especially the case within specific social contexts (e.g., parents sharing their own prescription drugs with their children to self-treat, college students using stimulants not prescribed to them to study). Part of this social acceptance is the idea that prescription drugs are safer than street drugs. Because prescription drugs are made by a pharmaceutical company, have a medical use, and are regulated by the government, there is a perception that negative consequences such as addiction are less likely to occur. This has to do with the idea that ingredients and dosages in prescription drugs are more reliable than street drugs. Route of administration is also important, as most people consume prescription drugs in pill form, which is a safer route of administration than snorting, smoking, or injection. There is also a perception that the use of prescription drugs will not produce an arrest or create a stigmatized identity. A person caught using pills is likely to be labeled as someone with a medical condition and not someone who simply wants to get high. Finally, prescription drugs are much more widely available compared to drugs such as heroin and cocaine. To acquire drugs such as heroin and cocaine generally involves contact with dealers in open-air street drug markets, while prescription drugs can be easily obtained from a doctor, family members, or friends.

Another important aspect is related to health and wellness. The conventional wisdom today is that there is a pill to help manage any physical or mental health problem a person has. We have embraced to motto "better living through chemistry," if you will. For example, high cholesterol is a medical condition faced by millions of Americans. High cholesterol is problematic because it is related to a number of negative health outcomes, including heart disease and stroke. We also know that high cholesterol is related to diet and levels of physical activity. Generally, high cholesterol is a problem for adults. So, let's say at 50 years old you are diagnosed with high cholesterol. You know the causes and the potential consequences, so what do you do? Do you try to change your eating and exercise habits, which have been in place for decades, or do you turn to a pill to lower your cholesterol? While this example focuses on a chronic physical condition that can be treated by a drug that will not get you high, the same logic can be used for more dangerous prescription drugs. We talked extensively in this chapter about the use of opioids to treat pain and how chronic pain was not an issue that doctors treated with opioids in the past. We can also talk about prescription benzodiazepines (e.g., Valium and Xanax) that can be used to treat people with mental health problems (e.g., anxiety, panic, insomnia).

It is important to talk about health and wellness, how more people are dealing with chronic pain and mental health issues, and how prescription drugs have become the go-to form of treatment. Much of this is related to what medical sociologists refer to as the sick role.[47] This is related to basic sociological concepts of status (a social position that a person occupies) and role (behavioral expectations that are attached to a status). The concept of status is easy to understand, as gender, race, educational level, marital status, and sickness are all statuses an individual can occupy. So the sick role simply outlines the behavioral expectations, or rights and obligations, that we have in our culture related to illness. Generally speaking, a person is not held as being responsible for being sick, and being sick allows the person to be exempt from social roles. For example, if a college student gets the flu and misses an exam, he or she is not blamed for the illness and is permitted to make up the missed assignment when he or she is feeling better. There is also an expectation that a sick person should make an attempt to get well and should seek help from medical professionals to facilitate this. In essence, when people get sick, we excuse them from normal activities but expect them to get better and return to social activities as soon as possible.

The sick role may help us understand the symbolic meaning that people attach to prescription drug misuse and how prescription drug misuse impacts their identity. Research shows that a significant portion of people who develop substance use disorders associated with prescription drug misuse initiate misuse due to a medical condition and a legal prescription from a doctor. Thus, they see themselves as patients in need of treatment and not addicts in need of a high. There are other reasons that the symbolic meaning associated with prescription drug misuse may be different than with traditional drug use. People may seek out prescription drugs because they view them as a safer alternative to street drugs. They have confidence in the ingredients because they were manufactured by a pharmaceutical company; they can be taken in pill form and do not have to be snorted, smoked, or injected; they are more readily available, which reduces the risk of arrest; and there is less stigma associated with use. All of this is related to identity, as people who use prescription drugs are seen as people with a medical condition, while people who use street drugs are viewed as people who want to get high.

Conclusion

This chapter outlined the whys to help understand how prescription drug misuse became the second most common type of drug use in the United States. It is important to understand the history of drug use in the United States. While we tend to view drug users as outsiders, this runs counter to the evidence that suggests that alcohol and drug use are a significant part of our culture. It is also important to understand the role of the medical-industrial complex, specifically how the treatment of pain changed over time. We discussed how the pharmaceutical industry used thought leaders and educational programs to convince doctors and patients that prescription opioids were safe and could be widely used to treat chronic pain. It is also important to review the academic literature on prescription drug misuse. To that end, we discussed theoretical explanations, correlates of misuse, and the importance of motives and sources. Research needs to identify how prescription drugs are different from other drugs, and we need to recognize that not all prescription drug misuse is the same. Finally, we discussed Golub's theory of subcultural evolution and used it to frame a discussion of the prescription drug era.

CHAPTER THREE

Middle-Class Prescription Medication Misuse and Diseases of Despair

Media portrayals of the prescription drug problem in the United States often paint a dire picture of rampant prescription drug misuse among middle-class suburbanites and wealthy Americans. Almost all of the high-profile media coverage of prescription drug misuse, addiction, and death is about celebrities or other well-to-do Americans. Chris Christie, the former governor of New Jersey and the chair of Donald Trump's President's Commission on Combating Drug Addiction and the Opioid Crisis, would frequently discuss the problems that one of his friends from law school had with prescription drug misuse. As reported by Vox, Christie "describes this friend as perfect—incredibly smart, with a successful law practice, with a beautiful and brilliant wife and kids, and both good looking *and* athletic."[1] His friend, however, was prescribed opioid painkillers to treat a back injury he developed from running, and the prescription grew into an addiction that cost Christie's friend his family, his home, his law practice, and eventually his life. Dead at the age of 52 from a drug overdose, Christie's friend epitomizes the tragic struggle with prescription drug misuse faced by middle- and upper-class Americans. It is stories such as that of Christie's friend that have been imprinted in the minds of Americans as the representation of the prescription drug problem in the United States. In contrast to the *routinization of caricature* of poor minorities in urban neighborhoods addicted to crack cocaine in the 1980s, the typical image associated with the prescription drug epidemic is the middle-class white suburban resident.

Based on the national data described in Chapter 1, there is no doubt that the demographics of the current prescription drug misuse problem are different from prior drug use crises. The gap in prescription drug misuse between white and black Americans, women and men, rural and urban residents, and older and younger Americans is much smaller for prescription drug misuse than marijuana and many forms of hard drug use. Are the media representations of the prescription drug crisis being a middle-class problem in the United States accurate? Has the prescription drug misuse problem hit the middle class harder than poor populations?

Middle-Class Prescription Drug Misuse Patterns

Measuring prescription drug misuse among middle-class Americans is difficult, mainly because there is a great deal of disagreement as to what income ranges count as being middle class. Further, the definitions of what it means to be middle class change over time with inflation and depend on how many people live within each household. For the purposes of showing the trends in middle-class prescription drug misuse, we once again rely on data from the National Survey on Drug Use and Health (NSDUH). Across all years between 1994 and 2014, the NSDUH measures yearly income in three categories: $0–$19,999, $20,000–$49,999, and $50,000 and above. In a 2016 report, Pew Charitable Trusts defined the middle class as having incomes between 67 percent and 200 percent of the national median income. In 1994, for instance, the median U.S. household income was $32,264, which means that middle-class families in 1994 earned between $21,616 and $64,528. In 2014 the median family income was $54,398, so middle-class families earned between $36,446 and $108,796 in 2014. Because the income ranges in the NSDUH are limited, we focus on the trends in prescription drug use among the group of people with family incomes above $50,000. Although not ideal, a $50,000 income is in the middle-class income range and reflects drug use patterns among more affluent Americans across the entire 20-year period, which is important for gaining a fuller understanding of the intense media and political attention on the current prescription drug crisis in the United States. The drug use patterns of more affluent middle-class Americans, defined in this chapter as yearly incomes of $50,000 or above, are compared to the drug use patterns of lower-income Americans, defined as annual incomes below $50,000.

As illustrated in Table 12, the 2014 data showed that overall, 20.1 percent of Americans reported having ever misused a prescription medication

Table 12. Drug Use Patterns by Income, 2014

	< $20,000	$20,000–$49,999	$50,000+
Prescription Drug Misuse			
Ever used	21.4%	19.9%	19.8%
Past-year use	7.5%	5.5%	4.7%
Past-month use	3.4%	2.3%	2.0%
Marijuana Use			
Ever used	42.2%	41.6%	46.6%
Past-year use	18.6%	13.7%	11.1%
Past-month use	12.1%	9.1%	6.6%
Hard Drug Use			
Ever used	22.3%	20.9%	22.8%
Past-year use	5.0%	3.5%	2.5%
Past-month use	1.7%	1.3%	0.9%
Prescription Painkiller Misuse			
Ever used	15.5%	14.0%	12.6%
Past-year use	5.3%	4.0%	3.1%
Past-month use	2.3%	1.6%	1.3%
Heroin Use			
Ever used	3.3%	1.9%	1.2%
Past-year use	0.8%	0.4%	0.2%
Past-month use	0.3%	0.2%	0.1%

Source: 2014 NSDUH.

in that year. The data also showed that the prescription drug misuse lifetime prevalence rates are remarkably similar by income, with all income groups separated by less than one percentage point. Having misused a prescription medication at least once during one's lifetime was therefore evenly distributed among the different income groups, with the middle class being only slightly less likely than lower-income Americans to report having ever misused a prescription medication in 2014.

The gap in prescription drug misuse by different income levels, however, is wider for past-year and past-month prevalence rates. Less affluent Americans are more likely than middle-class Americans to have reported recent prescription drug misuse. The lowest-income group in the United States was 1.6 times more likely to report past-year prescription drug misuse than middle-class Americans and 1.7 times more likely than middle-class Americans to report past-month prescription medication misuse in 2014. Although middle-class Americans were equally likely to report the misuse of prescription drugs at least once in their lifetime as lower-income Americans, middle-class Americans were less likely to continue abusing prescription drugs on a yearly or monthly basis than lower-income Americans. Compared to lower-income Americans, the middle class in the United States did not have a unique problem with prescription drug misuse in 2014.

Even though middle-class Americans misused prescription medications at a lower rate than lower-income Americans in 2014, it is possible that the middle class was overrepresented in prescription drug misuse patterns compared with the use of marijuana and hard drugs. The lifetime prevalence rates of marijuana and hard drug use, however, show that middle-class Americans were actually 1.1 times *more* likely to have used marijuana at least once in their lifetime than Americans with lower yearly incomes and were slightly more likely to report having ever used a hard drug in 2014. Middle-class Americans therefore were *more likely* than lower-income Americans to report lifetime marijuana and hard drug use in the 2014 data.

Similar to the patterns of prescription drug misuse over time that show that middle-class Americans are less likely than lower-income Americans to continue to misuse prescription medications on a yearly or monthly basis, middle-class Americans are also less likely to continue to regularly use marijuana or hard drugs than lower-income Americans. The 2014 data showed that past-year marijuana was 1.7 times more likely among the lowest-income group of Americans than among middle-class Americans. Similarly, the lowest-income group in the United States was twice as likely as middle-class Americans to report past-year hard drug use.

Past-month marijuana and hard drug use patterns by income also showed that middle-class Americans were less likely than lower-income Americans to report drug use in the past month. The lowest-income group of Americans was 1.8 more likely than the middle class to report past-month marijuana use and 1.8 times more likely than the middle class to report past-month hard drug use in 2014.

Taken together, when drug use patterns of the lowest-income Americans and middle-class Americans are directly compared, it is clear that middle-class Americans were more likely or equally likely to have at least experimented with all forms of drug use, including prescription drug misuse, than lower income Americans. The middle class, however, is less likely to continue all forms of drug use on a yearly or monthly basis. The past-month drug use data show that the middle class does have a marginally unique problem with prescription drug misuse compared with hard drug or marijuana use. The lowest-income group in the United States was 1.7 times more likely than the middle class to report past-month prescription drug misuse, but the lowest-income Americans were 1.8 times more likely than the middle class to report past-month marijuana or hard drug use in 2014. In short, the income gap in prescription drug misuse is slightly narrower than the income gap in marijuana and hard drug use.

Because the vast majority of media and political attention has been devoted specifically to opioid-based painkillers, it is also important to investigate whether the middle class in the United States has a unique problem with opiate medications. In 2014, the lowest-income Americans were 1.2 times more likely to report having ever misused a prescription painkiller, 1.7 times more likely to report having misused a prescription painkiller in the past year, and 1.8 times more likely to report having misused a prescription painkiller in the past month than middle-class Americans. The income gap in prescription painkiller misuse is therefore strikingly similar to the income gap in overall prescription drug misuse.

To the small degree that prescription drug misuse is a larger problem among the middle class in the United States than marijuana or hard drug use, the problem is also reflected in the patterns of prescription painkiller misuse. Stated differently, like overall prescription drug misuse, prescription painkiller misuse is only a slightly bigger problem than other forms of drug use among middle-class Americans than among lower-income Americans. Although the transition from prescription painkiller misuse to heroin use among the middle class will be examined in detail later in this chapter, it is first important to examine the patterns of heroin use by income in 2014. In the 2014 data, the lowest-income group in the United States was 2.8 times more likely to report ever having used heroin than the middle class. Importantly, only a small percentage of Americans, regardless of income, reported having ever used heroin (1.2 percent of the middle class, 3.4 percent of the lowest-income group in the United States), much lower percentages than for other forms of drug use. Even fewer Americans reported past-year or past-month heroin use in the 2014 data, but again, the lowest-income Americans were 4 times more likely to report past-year heroin use and 3 times more likely to report past-month heroin use than middle-class Americans. Only 0.1 percent of middle-class Americans and 0.2 percent and 0.3 percent of lower-income Americans reported past-month heroin use in 2014. Heroin use is much more strongly concentrated among lower-income Americans than middle-class Americans. Additionally, prescription painkiller misuse was much more likely among all income groups than heroin use in 2014—past-month prescription painkiller misuse was 6.8 times more likely among the lowest-income group and 10.6 times more likely among middle-class Americans than past-month heroin use.

Trends in Prescription Drug Misuse among the Middle-Class from 1994 to 2014

The data described above shows that prescription drug misuse is only slightly more heavily concentrated among middle-class Americans than other forms of drug use. Lower-income Americans are much more likely than middle-class Americans to misuse all types of drugs, but the income difference in usage rates for prescription drug misuse was slightly smaller for prescription drugs than for marijuana or hard drugs. The patterns of drug misuse by income in 2014, however, do not tell the whole story of the prescription drug misuse problem in the United States. It is also important to understand trends in prescription drug misuse over the past 20 years to determine if the growth in prescription drug misuse among the middle class in the United States was more rapid than among other income groups during this period.

As shown in Table 13, past-month prescription drug misuse was slightly more common among the lowest-income group in the United States than among middle-class Americans in 1994. Between 1994 and 1998, the lowest-income group experienced a decline in prescription drug misuse, and the other two income groups, including middle-class Americans, both experienced rapid increases in prescription drug misuse. By 1998, prescription drug misuse was slightly more prevalent among the higher-income group than the lowest-income group in the United States. Past-month prescription drug misuse decreased among middle-class Americans from 1999 to 2001 but increased among lower-income Americans. In 2001, past-month prescription drug misuse was 1.8 times more common among the lowest-income group than among the middle class. From 2002 to 2014 the prescription drug misuse prevalence rate decreased for all income groups, but the decrease was more noticeable among the lower-income groups than middle-class Americans. The result of these patterns is that the income gap in prescription drug misuse increased slightly over the past 20 years, with the lowest-income group being 1.6 times more likely to report past-month prescription drug misuse in 1994 and 1.7 times more likely to report past-month prescription drug misuse in 2014.

Prescription drug misuse did not increase more rapidly among the middle class in the United States than the lower-income groups over the past 20 years, but recent data show that decreases in prescription drug misuse have been slower among the middle class than among the lower-income groups of Americans. The fact that the middle class was *also* affected by the growing prescription drug misuse crisis, however, is noteworthy and distinguishes the current prescription drug misuse problem as being unique in comparison to prior drug scares.

Table 13. Past-Month Drug Use Patterns by Income, 1994–2014

	< $20,000	$20,000–$49,999	$50,000+
Prescription Drug Misuse			
% Change 1994–1998	–15.5% (0.71%–0.60%)	91.7% (0.36%–0.69%)	45.5% (0.44%–0.64%)
% Change 1999–2001	21.3% (2.35%–2.85%)	51.1% (1.31%–1.98%)	–0.6% (1.60%–1.59%)
% Change 2002–2014	–15.4% (3.97%–3.36%)	–7.2% (2.49%–2.31%)	–3.0% (2.02%–1.96%)
Marijuana Use			
% Change 1994–1998	36.5% (3.12%–4.26%)	93.3% (1.78%–3.44%)	53.0% (2.30%–3.52%)
% Change 1999–2001	4.3% (6.28%–6.55%)	15.5% (4.70%–5.43%)	29.9% (3.41%–4.43%)
% Change 2002–2014	56.2% (7.72%–12.06%)	41.4% (6.42%–9.08%)	28.5% (5.12%–6.58%)
Hard Drug Use			
% Change 1994–1998	10.0% (0.90%–0.99%)	46.7% (0.45%–0.66%)	77.6% (0.49%–0.87%)
% Change 1999–2001	21.0% (1.62%–1.96%)	23.1% (1.04%–1.28%)	1.1% (0.95%–0.96%)
% Change 2002–2014	–30.4% (2.40%–1.67%)	0.8% (1.26%–1.27%)	–22.5% (1.20%–0.93%)
Prescription Painkiller Misuse			
% Change 1994–1998	2.6% (0.39%–0.40%)	152.4% (0.21%–0.53%)	47.1% (0.34%–0.50%)
% Change 1999–2001	52.2% (1.36%–2.07%)	53.2% (0.94%–1.44%)	–0.9% (1.14%–1.13%)
% Change 2002–2014	–16.5% (2.78%–2.32%)	–1.8% (1.66%–1.63%)	–16.4% (1.52%–1.27%)
Heroin Use			
% Change 1994–1998	–70.4% (0.27%–0.08%)	inf. (0.00%–0.01%)	inf. (0.00%–0.06%)
% Change 1999–2001	22.2% (0.09%–0.11%)	0.0% (0.05%–0.05%)	–40.0% (0.05%–0.03%)
% Change 2002–2014	88.9% (0.18%–0.34%)	650.0% (0.02%–0.15%)	71.4% (0.07%–0.12%)

Source: 1994–2014 NSDUH.

In contrast to the uneven development of the prescription drug misuse problem in the United States, whereby each income group experienced increases and decreases in the prevalence of prescription drug misuse over the past 20 years, marijuana use increased among all income groups in each period over the past 20 years. Like prescription drug misuse, the income gap in past-month marijuana use also increased over the past 20 years. In 1994 past-month marijuana use was 1.4 times more likely among the lowest-income group compared to middle-class Americans, but by 2014 the lowest-income group was 1.8 times more likely to report past-month marijuana use than middle-class Americans. Although marijuana use increased among all income groups in the United States since 1994, the increases were more rapid among the lowest-income group.

Hard drug use prevalence rates by income over the past 20 years show that past-month hard drug use increased more rapidly among the middle class in the early part of the period investigated, but past-month hard drug use increased more slowly than the lower-income groups from 1999 to 2001. The hard drug use prevalence rate decreased substantially among the lowest-income group and among the middle class from 2002 to 2014, but past-month hard drug use increased slightly among the $20,000–$49,999 income group. Like prescription drug misuse and marijuana use, despite a slight narrowing of the income gap in hard drug use in the late 1990s and early 2000s, the lowest-income Americans were 1.8 times more likely than the middle class to report past-month hard drug use in both 1994 and 2014.

Overall, the middle class in the United States was not more strongly affected by the growing prescription drug crisis than either of the lower-income groups over the past 20 years. The best conclusion that can be made from this data is that the income gap in all forms of drug use narrowed slightly in the late 1990s and early 2000s, but the income gap in all forms of drug use returned to the same level in 2014 as it was in 1994. It should also be noted, however, that from 2002 to 2014, the decreases in prescription drug misuse among the middle class were much slower than among the lower-income groups, a finding that suggests that the U.S. middle class has been more reluctant than the lower-income groups to abandon prescription drug misuse.

Although the income gap in overall prescription drug misuse did not narrow substantially over the past 20 years, the data do show that the U.S. middle class has had at different times a unique problem with opioid misuse, whether in the form of prescription painkiller misuse or heroin use. Between 1994 and 1998, the prescription painkiller misuse prevalence rate increased rapidly among the middle class but only increased very slowly among the lowest-income Americans. The past-month prescription painkiller misuse rate more than doubled among Americans earning between $20,000 and $49,999 during this same period. By 1998, middle-class Americans were 1.3 times more likely to report past-month prescription painkiller misuse than the lowest-income group in the United States. Between 1999 and 2001, however, middle-class Americans experienced a slight decrease in the prevalence of prescription painkiller misuse, but the lower-income groups experienced further increases in the prevalence of prescription painkiller misuse. By 2001 the lowest-income group in the United States showed the highest past-month prescription painkiller misuse rate, 1.8 times greater than the middle-class prevalence rate. Declines in past-month prescription painkiller misuse occurred between 2002 and 2014 for all income groups, but the rate of decline was faster among the lowest-income group and the middle class than the $20,000–$49,999 group, which showed only a small decline. Across this period between 2002 and 2014, however, the lowest-income Americans remained 1.8 times more likely than the middle class to report past-month prescription painkiller misuse. Prescription painkiller misuse was a bigger problem among the middle class than the lower-income groups at the beginning of the prescription drug misuse problem in the United States, but the lower-income groups quickly embraced prescription painkiller misuse and are now more likely than the middle class to misuse these analgesic medications.

Past-month heroin use was quite rare in all periods over the past 20 years, especially among the middle class. Essentially, no middle-class Americans reported past-month heroin use in 1994. Between 1994 and 1998, heroin use entered the higher-income groups during a period when the lowest-income Americans experienced substantial increases in past-month heroin use. By 1998, the lowest-income Americans were 1.3 times more likely than the middle class to report past-month heroin use. Increases in past-month heroin use occurred among the lowest-income Americans from 1999 to 2001, when the middle-class experienced a decrease in past-month heroin use rates. Most strikingly, past-month heroin use spiked in all income groups in the United States between 2002 and 2014. Past-month heroin use increased by 71 percent in the middle class, 650 percent in the $20,000–$49,999 group, and 89 percent in the lowest-income group during this period. By 2014 the lowest-income group in the United States was 2.8 times more likely than the middle class to report past-month heroin use, but the fact that the middle class experienced substantial increases in heroin use over the past 20 years, especially since 2002, is noteworthy nonetheless.

From Pill Popping to Shooting Up?

Despite the relative rarity of heroin use in the United States, the media has featured countless stories of middle-class Americans who started experimenting with prescription opioid medications as recreational drugs and eventually turned to heroin. A recent CNN article titled "Inside the Secret Lives of Functioning Heroin Addicts," for instance, highlights several middle- and upper-class people who live with secret heroin addictions and continue to live outwardly normal lives.[2] One of the subjects featured in the story, who goes by the pseudonym Tom in the article and works in a high-income corporate management career, was a typical suburban high school student who occasionally used marijuana but took a Percocet that his mother left lying around his house after a surgery and became addicted. He now misuses prescription opioids but will use heroin when prescription opioids are too expensive or otherwise not available. Another person featured in the article who goes by the name Lisa was an excellent student in a college-prep high school, currently works in retail management, and has a strong and supportive marriage. Lisa began using opioid medications to treat knee and back problems. But when state and local governments began regulating legal prescriptions for opioid medications, she turned to illegal prescription opioids. The illegal prescription opioids, however, became too expensive, so Lisa turned to heroin.

Stories such as these of middle-class Americans turning away from prescription opioid misuse and toward heroin are all too common in mainstream media accounts of the current drug misuse crisis. But does research support that this trend is occurring and/or escalating among the middle class in the United States? Prior research has clearly shown that the nonmedical use of prescription opioids is a risk factor for heroin use[3] and that recent trends in people seeking treatment for heroin addiction are increasingly likely to be middle class, white, and living in nonurban areas.[4] Furthermore, Compton and colleagues report that the overall trend in prescription opioid misusers who also use heroin has increased substantially in recent years. Christopher Jones additionally shows that the likelihood of heroin misuse is 40 times greater for people who misuse prescription opioids than for people who do not misuse prescription opioid medications.[5] This research clearly points to a major and growing trend in Americans transitioning from prescription opioid misuse to heroin use.

As alarming as the prior research connecting prescription opioid misuse and heroin use appears, the percentage of prescription opioid misusers who turn to heroin use is actually quite small. As Compton and associates state, "although the majority of current heroin users report having used prescription opioids nonmedically before they initiated heroin use, heroin use among people who use prescription opioids for nonmedical reasons is rare, and the transition to heroin use appears to occur at a low rate."[6] Research has established that only 3.6 percent of prescription opioid misusers began using heroin within five years of beginning prescription opioid misuse. Additionally, as we reported in an earlier chapter, only .08 percent of the U.S. population reported abusing any prescription drug alongside any hard drug in 2014. Given the relatively large numbers of prescription opioid misusers in the United States, however, it must be noted that even small shifts toward heroin among this group of prescription opioid misusers translates into tens of thousands of new heroin users.

The greatest risk of transitioning from prescription opioid misuse to heroin use is among the subgroup of very high-rate nonmedical opioid users. Jones reports that "Among past year nonmedical users, the highest rate of past year heroin use was found among frequent nonmedical users—people reporting 100–365 days of PYNMU [past-year nonmedical use]."[7] Importantly, among this group of high-rate prescription opioid misusers, 83 percent reported abusing opioid medications prior to using heroin, and the rate of abusing prescription opioids prior to initiating heroin use has increased in recent years. Even among the high-rate prescription opioid misusers, however, only 9.5 percent also reported heroin use. High-rate prescription opioid misuse is clearly a risk factor for heroin use, but the rate of transitioning to heroin use is quite small.

Overall, prior research suggests that prescription opioid misuse is associated with heroin use in the United States even if the percentages of people transitioning from opioid medication misuse to heroin use is minimal. But no prior research has specifically examined the patterns of transitioning from opioid medication misuse to heroin use by income level. To assess the degree to which past-month prescription painkiller misuse develops into past-month heroin use for each income group, we once again rely on data from the NSDUH. Specifically, we calculate year-by-year percentage changes in the prevalence of both past-year painkiller misuse and heroin use for each income group to determine the degree to which changes in one form of drug use are associated with changes in the other form of drug use from 2002 to 2014.

The patterns of prescription opioid misuse and heroin use patterns by income groups are shown in Table 14. The first evidence of moves away from prescription opioid misuse and toward heroin use is shown in the years when past-month prescription painkiller misuse declined and past-month heroin use increased. For the lowest-income group, prescription

Table 14. Prescription Painkiller and Heroin Misuse Trends, 2002–2014

	<$20,000		$20,000–$49,999		$50,000+	
	Pres. Pain	Heroin	Pres. Pain	Heroin	Pres. Pain	Heroin
2002–2003	–6.1%	–44.4%	7.2%	100.0%	16.6%	–42.9%
2003–2004	–11.5%	20.0%	2.2%	100.0%	–9.6%	–25.0%
2004–2005	13.0%	–25.0%	5.5%	–25.0%	–6.6%	0.0%
2005–2006	4.2%	244.4%	–3.6%	83.3%	14.7%	133.3%
2006–2007	–5.1%	–71.0%	20.0%	–27.3%	–6.7%	–57.1%
2007–2008	–1.6%	33.3%	–12.6%	50.0%	1.2%	100.0%
2008–2009	20.9%	66.7%	12.4%	–25.0%	–3.2%	–50.0%
2009–2010	–15.0%	–20.0%	–3.7%	–33.3%	0.5%	200.0%
2010–2011	–5.0%	56.3%	–11.9%	–16.7%	–18.2%	–11.1%
2011–2012	–14.1%	8.0%	11.9%	100.0%	21.6%	–12.5%
2012–2013	18.3%	–7.4%	–14.0%	–20.0%	–14.8%	–14.3%
2013–2014	–7.9%	36.0%	–8.4%	87.5%	–9.1%	100.0%
2002–2014	–16.5%	88.9%	–1.8%	650.0%	–16.4%	71.4%

Source: 1994–2014 NSDUH.

painkiller misuse prevalence rates declined and heroin use prevalence rates increased in 5 of the 12 transition years between 2002 and 2014. For the group who earned between $20,000 and $49,999, the pattern of prescription painkiller misuse declining and heroin use increasing occurred in 3 of the 12 transition years studied. Among those who earned more than $50,000 per year, prescription painkiller misuse declined and heroin use increased in only 1 transition year, 2013–2014. Importantly, prescription painkiller misuse rates decreased and heroin use rates increased for all income groups in only one period, 2013–2014, the most recent period available in the NSDUH data.

Just as years when prescription painkiller misuse declined and heroin use increased is of interest to understanding the relationship between heroin and prescription opioids, so is the opposite situation, when prescription painkiller misuse rates increased and heroin use rates declined. This occurred in 2 of the 12 transition years for the lowest-income Americans, 3 of the 12 transition years for the $20,000–$49,999 group, and only 1 of the transition years for higher-income Americans. Overall, a simple look at the prescription painkiller misuse and heroin use patterns by income suggests that the transition from prescription opioid misuse to heroin use is more likely among lower-income Americans than among middle-class Americans.

From 2002 to 2012, however, all income groups did show overall declines in the prevalence of prescription painkiller and increases in the prevalence of heroin use. Prescription opioid misuse and heroin use are clearly related. The correlation between past-year prescription painkiller misuse and past-year heroin use over the 12 years in this analysis is −0.20 for the lowest-income Americans and −0.29 for the highest-income Americans. This means that as prescription painkiller misuse decreases heroin use tends to increase for the low- and high-income groups, and that trend is slightly stronger among the middle class than among lower-income Americans. Interestingly, the correlation between prescription painkiller misuse and heroin use among the $20,000–$49,999 group of Americans is 0.05, which suggests that there is a very weak positive association between past-year prescription painkiller misuse and past-year heroin use among this group; as prescription opioid misuse increases, so does heroin use among this income group. This relationship, however, is very weak. The best conclusion from this data is that the transition from prescription painkiller misuse to heroin use is occurring most strongly among the lowest-income group in the United States, but there is certainly some evidence that this drug use pattern is also occurring among middle-class Americans, especially in the most recent years.

The sheer numbers of people in the United States who transition from prescription painkiller misuse to heroin use are also important to analyze to gain a fuller picture of this problem. Among middle-class Americans, prescription painkiller misuse decreased by 16 percent from 2002 to 2014. In 2002, 1.52 percent of this group reported past-month prescription painkiller misuse, which reduced to 1.27 percent of this group in 2014. Across this period, 0.25 percent fewer middle-class Americans were past-month prescription painkiller misusers in 2014 than in 2002. Based on the number of middle-class Americans in the United States in 2014, the change in prescription painkiller misuse from 2002 to 2014 equates to 338,000 fewer middle-class prescription opioid misusers in 2014 compared to 2002. Using the same calculation for the increase in past-month heroin use among the middle class in the United States over this same period, there were approximately 67,000 more middle-class past-month heroin users in 2014 than in 2002. For every 5 middle-class Americans who stopped abusing prescription painkillers between 2002 and 2014, 1 middle-class American began using heroin.

Among the lowest-income Americans, the decrease in past-month prescription painkiller misuse from 2002 to 2014 equates to 221,000 fewer low-income American prescription painkiller misusers in 2014 than in 2002. The increase in past-month heroin use among the lowest-income group of Americans equates to 77,000 more low-income Americans being regular heroin users in 2014 than in 2002. For every 3 low-income Americans who stopped abusing prescription painkillers between 2002 and 2014, 1 low-income American began using heroin.

Among Americans with yearly incomes between $20,000 and $49,999, the patterns of prescription drug misuse and heroin use are more complicated. Overall, this group experienced a slight reduction in the prevalence of past-month prescription painkiller misuse between 2002 and 2014, which equates to a reduction of approximately 24,000 prescription painkiller misusers in this income group between 2002 and 2014. In contrast, past-month heroin use among this group increased dramatically (650 percent) between 2002 and 2014, a change that equates to approximately 106,000 more past-month heroin users in this income group in 2014 than in 2002. For every American with a yearly income between $20,000 and $49,999 who stopped abusing prescription painkillers between 2002 and 2014, more than 4 Americans in this income range began using heroin. In other words, more Americans in this income group began using heroin between 2002 and 2014 than stopped abusing prescription painkillers.

Based on prior research and the current analysis, there is clearly an association between prescription opioid misuse and heroin use, and it appears that the connection has become stronger in recent years. Rates of prescription painkiller misuse decreased substantially from 2013 to 2014 for all income groups, but the decrease was slightly larger among middle-class Americans than lower-income Americans. During this time heroin use rates rose significantly for all groups, but again, the increase in heroin use was more substantial for the middle-class. Between 2013 and 2014 alone, the middle class in the United States added 81,000 heroin users and lost 40,000 prescription painkiller misusers. With a total of 1.7 million middle-class past-month prescription painkiller misusers and 81,000 middle-class past-month heroin users in 2014, it is clear that the middle class has an opioid problem that is beginning to shift from prescription painkillers to heroin.

In comparison, however, the lowest-income Americans added 43,000 heroin users and lost 96,000 prescription painkiller misusers from 2013 to 2014. The lowest-income group included a total of 1.1 million past-month prescription painkiller misusers and 163,000 past-month heroin users in 2014. The group of Americans with yearly incomes between $20,000 and $49,999 lost 122,000 past-month prescription painkiller misusers and added 57,000 heroin users between 2013 and 2014. There were a total of 1.9 million prescription painkiller misusers and 278,000 heroin users among this group in 2014. This shows that the middle class, in raw numbers, added more heroin users and lost fewer prescription painkiller misusers than either of the lower-income groups between 2013 and 2014.

More than one-third of all prescription opioid misusers were middle-class Americans in 2014, while only 15 percent of the total decrease in prescription opioid misusers between 2013 and 2014 were middle-class Americans. The middle class also accounted for 15.5 percent of all heroin users in 2014 but accounted 22 percent of the increase in heroin users from 2013 to 2014. These trends set the stage for even greater problems with both prescription opioid misuse and heroin use for the middle class in the future.

Conclusion

The overall trend away from prescription opioid misuse and toward heroin use among the middle class in the United States shown in the data presented above provides some support to the public view that middle-class prescription painkiller misusers are transitioning to heroin for their opioid fixes. Although the negative correlation between prescription opioid and heroin use is stronger among the middle class than the lower-income groups across the 12-year period between 2002 and 2014, the lowest-income Americans experienced the largest overall decline in prescription painkiller misuse and the highest overall increase in heroin use. The transition away from prescription painkillers and toward heroin therefore occurred at a more rapid pace among the lowest-income group in the United States than among the middle class during this period. More distressingly, the group of Americans with incomes between $20,000 and $49,999 experienced a much larger increase in the number of heroin users than the group lost in prescription opioid misusers. Heroin is quickly infiltrating that income group in the United States without reductions in the number of prescription painkiller misusers. Although firm conclusions are not possible with the NSDUH data presented, it is clear that some of the lowest-income and middle-class Americans who stopped abusing prescription opiates moved on to become heroin users, but prior research on the topic suggests that the number of people who transition from prescription opioid misuse to heroin use is quite small.

The other distressing conclusion from the data presented above is that the middle class added twice as many heroin users between 2013 and 2014 than were lost in prescription opioid misusers. It appears that the middle class is adopting heroin use at a higher rate rather than abandoning prescription opioid use. Heroin is beginning to intrude into the U.S. middle class, prior prescription painkiller abuse or not, although the percentage of past-month heroin users among the middle class remains lower than the percentage of past-month heroin users in the lower-income groups in the United States. The most recent data therefore do not fully support that heroin use among the middle class stemmed primarily from prescription opioid misuse. Among lower-income Americans, however, both groups lost more prescription opioid misuser than were gained in heroin users, which suggests that at least in the most recent data available, the transition from prescription opioid misuse to heroin use is stronger among lower-income Americans.

To the degree that public policies have increased the black market prices of prescription opioid medications, as is consistently stressed in media depictions of the current drug problem, it makes sense that the transition from prescription opioid misuse to heroin is more highly concentrated among lower-income groups than among the middle class. The Drug Enforcement Administration reported that in markets where both heroin and illicit prescription opioids are available, prices for heroin were always lower, and heroin has increased in purity in recent years.[8] A bag of heroin, for instance, sells for about $10, whereas an illicit prescription opioid pill sells for about $20 on the black market,[9] and the high from heroin is much stronger. The introduction of fentanyl into heroin markets has further increased the potency of heroin and dramatically reduced the cost.[10] Fentanyl is substantially more potent than heroin and is manufactured in illegal markets for a fraction of the price of heroin. There is therefore a financial incentive for heroin distributors to lace the product with fentanyl, and the decreased price and increased potency of fentanyl-laced heroin provides a financial incentive for opioid misusers to use heroin instead. For lower-income Americans who are dependent on opioids, addictions that usually begin with prescription opioids, transitioning from the more expensive opioid medications to the less expensive heroin is financially sensible. For middle-class Americans with greater access to financial resources, continuing to misuse prescription opioids, even if more expensive than heroin, is more likely due to the stigma that surrounds heroin use.

Is Prescription Drug Misuse an Issue among Middle-Class Women?

In the early part of the 20th century, women were portrayed as the first group to misuse prescription medications in a widespread way, and there has been some concern expressed that women, specifically middle-class women, have driven the prescription drug misuse problem. In 2014, 2.1 percent of middle-class males reported past-year prescription drug misuse, whereas 1.9 percent of middle-class women reported the same past-year prescription drug misuse; middle-class men were only slightly more than middle-class women likely to report past-month prescription drug misuse. Compared with other drugs, however, middle-class women are more highly represented in prescription drug misuse than marijuana or hard drug use. To illustrate, the 2014 data displayed in Table 15 show that middle-class men were 1.8 times more likely to use marijuana and 2.4 times more likely to report past-month hard drug use than middle-class women. Focusing specifically on opioids, middle-class men were 1.9 times more likely to report past-month heroin use but only 1.4 times more likely to report past-month prescription painkiller use than middle-class women in 2014. The conclusion that can be drawn from this data is that although middle-class males are more likely to report past-month prescription drug misuse than middle-class women, the middle-class gender gap in prescription drug misuse is much smaller than the middle-class gender gap for marijuana or hard drug use. Therefore, middle-class women do have a unique problem with prescription drug misuse compared to middle-class men.

The trends in prescription drug misuse over time among middle-class men and women shown in Table 15 are also important in understanding the prescription drug misuse problem among middle-class Americans. In 1994, a slightly greater percentage of middle-class women reported past-month prescription drug misuse than middle-class men, but between 1994 and 1998, the prescription drug misuse rate increased more rapidly among middle-class men than among middle-class women. Slight declines in the prescription drug misuse rate occurred between 1999 and 2001 for both middle-class men and women, but between 2002 and 2014 the prescription drug misuse rate for middle-class women decreased slightly and remained stable for middle-class men. For most of the past 20 years, a slightly higher percentage of middle-class men reported past-month prescription drug misuse than middle-class women, but in two years (2000 and 2012), the percentage of middle-class women who misused prescription drugs slightly exceeded the percentage of middle-class men who reported past-month prescription drug misuse.

In contrast to the trends in prescription drug misuse over the past 20 years, where the prevalence increases were smaller and decreases were more pronounced among middle-class women than men, the past-month marijuana use rates increased more rapidly among middle-class women than men in all periods between 1994 and 2014. Further, although hard drug use is much less common among middle-class women than men in

Table 15. Past-Month Middle-Class Drug Use Patterns by Sex and Race, 1994–2014

	Males	Females	Whites	Minorities
Prescription Drug Misuse				
% Change 1994–1998	114.0%	34.8%	38.0%	147.1%
	(0.43%–0.92%)	(0.46%–0.62%)	(0.50%–0.69%)	(0.17%–0.42%)
% Change 1999–2001	−0.6%	−2.0%	−4.6%	31.9%
	(1.70%–1.69%)	(1.50%–1.47%)	(1.75%–1.67%)	(0.91%–1.20%)
% Change 2002–2014	0.0%	−5.6%	−10.3%	33.5%
	(2.07%–2.07%)	(1.96%–1.85%)	(2.13%–1.91%)	(1.58%–2.11%)
Marijuana Use				
% Change 1994–1998	61.1%	201.1%	67.2%	−42.8%
	(3.24%–5.22%)	(0.95%–2.86%)	(1.90%–3.74%)	(4.11%–2.35%)
% Change 1999–2001	18.6%	52.3%	27.0%	44.3%
	(4.56%–5.41%)	(2.20%–3.35%)	(3.45%–4.38%)	(3.23%–4.66%)
% Change 2002–2014	24.0%	39.4%	27.3%	47.0%
	(6.75%–8.37%)	(3.35%–4.67%)	(5.42%–6.90%)	(3.89%–5.72%)
Hard Drug Use				
% Change 1994–1998	105.1%	61.8%	77.4%	66.7%
	(0.59%–1.21%)	(0.34%–0.55%)	(0.53%–0.94%)	(0.30%–0.50%)
% Change 1999–2001	−10.0%	23.7%	2.1%	−5.7%
	(1.30%–1.17%)	(0.59%–0.73%)	(0.97%–0.99%)	(0.87%–0.82%)
% Change 2002–2014	−23.7%	−19.4%	−26.1%	−17.5%
	(1.69%–1.29%)	(0.67%–0.54%)	(1.15%–0.85%)	(1.37%–1.13%)

Prescription Painkiller Misuse				
% Change 1994–1998	41.9% (0.43%–0.61%)	128.6% (0.21%–0.48%)	40.5% (0.37%–0.52%)	129.4% (0.17%–0.39%)
% Change 1999–2001	2.4% (1.24%–1.27%)	–5.8% (1.03%–0.97%)	–5.7% (1.23%–1.16%)	40.0% (0.70%–0.98%)
% Change 2002–2014	–11.6% (1.64%–1.45%)	–23.6% (1.40%–1.07%)	–25.6% (1.60%–1.19%)	22.5% (1.20%–1.47%)
Heroin Use				
% Change 1994–1998	inf. (0.00%–0.0.04%)	inf. (0.00%–0.03%)	inf. (0.00%–0.07%)	inf. (0.00%–0.01%)
% Change 1999–2001	–62.5% (0.08%–0.03%)	–33.3% (0.03%–0.02%)	0.0% (0.02%–0.02%)	–68.4% (0.19%–0.06%)
% Change 2002–2014	25.0% (0.12%–0.15%)	700.0% (0.01%–0.08%)	100.0% (0.07%–0.14%)	–14.3% (0.07%–0.06%)

Source: 1994–2014 NSDUH.

all periods over the past 20 years, the gender gap in middle-class drug misuse has decreased in recent years. From 1999 to 2001, the past-month hard drug use rate increased among middle-class women but decreased among middle-class men. Additionally, the hard drug use prevalence rate decreased more slowly between 2002 and 2014 among middle-class women than among men.

Prescription painkiller misuse evolved differently among middle-class men and women over the past 20 years than general prescription drug misuse. Prescription painkiller misuse was twice as likely among middle-class men than women in 1994, but the more substantial increase in prescription painkiller misuse among middle-class women between 1994 and 1998 resulted in a narrowing of the gender gap in prescription painkiller misuse. By 1998, middle-class men were only slightly more likely to report past-month prescription painkiller misuse than middle-class women. A small increase in prescription painkiller misuse occurred among middle-class men from 1999 to 2001, a time in which prescription painkiller misuse declined slightly among middle-class women. Large decreases in prescription painkiller misuse occurred between 2002 and 2014 for all middle-class Americans, but the rate of decrease was more substantial for middle-class women than for men. Overall, after the large increase in past-month prescription painkiller misuse among middle-class women between 1994 and 1998, prescription drug misuse remained 1.2 to 1.3 times more likely among middle-class men than among middle-class women.

Heroin use was essentially nonexistent among middle-class men and women in 1994, but by 1998, 0.04 percent of middle-class men and 0.03 percent of middle-class women reported past-month heroin use. Heroin use decreased among middle-class men and women from 1999 to 2001, but only a small fraction of the middle class was using heroin across this period too. Although heroin use remained rare among the middle class between 2002 and 2014, past-month heroin use rates increased during this period for middle-class men and women. Most notably, however, middle-class women showed a 700 percent increase in past-month heroin use between 2002 and 2014, whereas middle-class men showed only a 25 percent increase. As distressing as the percentage increase among middle-class women appears, middle-class men were nearly twice as likely as women to report past-month heroin use in 2014. Because past-month prescription painkiller misuse decreased by 24 percent among middle-class women between 2002 and 2014, the rapid increase in past-month heroin use among middle-class women is evidence that the transition from prescription painkiller misuse to heroin has likely occurred at a more rapid pace among middle-class women in recent years. A much smaller decrease in prescription painkiller misuse and a much smaller increase in heroin use occurred among middle-class men during this same period.

Middle-class women clearly have a unique problem with prescription drug misuse, including prescription painkiller misuse, evidenced by the data showing a much narrower gender gap in the middle class for prescription drug misuse than for other forms of drug use. Although prescription painkiller misuse prevalence rates have declined in recent years for middle-class males and females, the most recent data also raise serious concerns about a rapid increase in heroin use among middle-class women. The prevalence of heroin use remains very low among middle-class women, with prescription painkiller misuse being more than 13 times more likely than heroin use in 2014 among middle-class women, but the data indicate that some middle-class women who abandon prescription painkiller misuse are beginning to turn to heroin instead.

Is Prescription Drug Abuse an Issue among Middle-Class White Americans?

Another factor driving public and political concern about the prescription drug misuse crisis in the United States is the impression that middle-class whites are disproportionately impacted by this growing problem. As with the discussion of middle-class men and women above, the 2014 data show that middle-class minorities in the United States misuse prescription medications at a higher rate than middle-class whites, but the middle-class race gap in prescription drug use is smaller for prescription drug misuse than some other drugs. As shown in Table 14, middle-class minorities were 1.1 times more likely than middle-class whites to report past-month prescription drug misuse in 2014. Because middle-class minorities were 1.3 times more likely to report past-month hard drug use in 2014, the middle-class race gap in prescription drug misuse was smaller than the race gap in hard drug use in that year. In contrast, however, middle-class whites are actually 1.2 times *more* likely than middle-class minorities to report past-month marijuana use. This means that the middle-class race gap was narrower for prescription drug misuse than hard drug use, thereby indicating that prescription drug misuse was more of a problem among middle-class whites than other drugs, but middle-class whites were using marijuana at a much higher rate than middle-class minorities.

Patterns of opioid misuse among middle-class whites and minorities further highlight the unique nature of the current prescription drug problem in the United States. The race gap in prescription painkiller misuse among the middle class, for instance, is wider than the race gap among the middle class for prescription drug misuse as a whole. Middle-class minorities were 1.3 times more likely than middle-class whites to report past-month prescription painkiller misuse in 2014. Middle-class whites, in contrast, were 2.3 more likely than middle-class minorities to report past-month heroin use in 2014.

Is prescription drug misuse a unique problem among middle-class white Americans? The answer is yes. Compared with hard drug use patterns among the middle class by race, middle-class whites are slightly overrepresented among prescription drug misusers. On the other hand, marijuana and heroin use are much bigger problems among middle-class whites than middle-class minorities.

The trends in prescription drug misuse over time paint a more precise picture of the racial dynamics involved in drug misuse by race among the middle class in the United States. In 1994, past-month prescription drug misuse was three times more likely among middle-class white Americans than among middle-class minorities, but prescription drug misuse rates rose much more rapidly among middle-class minorities over the period from 1994 to 1998. By 1998, middle-class whites were only 1.6 times more likely than middle-class minorities to report past-month prescription drug misuse. Between 1999 and 2001, the prescription drug misuse prevalence rate continued to increase among middle-class minorities but declined slightly among middle-class whites. The same pattern was shown between 2002 and 2014, when prescription drug misuse became more prevalent among middle-class minorities but less prevalent among middle-class whites. Prescription drug misuse began as a middle-class white American problem, but declines in prescription drug misuse among whites and increases in prescription drug misuse among minorities over the past 20 years have resulted in a shift in the racial patterns of prescription drug misuse. In 2014, a greater percentage of middle-class minorities reported past-month misuse of prescription drugs than middle-class whites.

The racial trends in middle-class marijuana use show a contrasting pattern to prescription drug misuse. Marijuana use was twice as likely among middle-class minorities as middle-class whites in 1994, but a large increase in past-month marijuana use among middle-class whites and a sharp decrease in past-month marijuana use among middle-class minorities between 1994 and 1998 resulted in whites being about 60 percent more likely to report past-month marijuana use in 1998. Although past-month marijuana use prevalence rates increased more rapidly among middle-class minorities in the 1999–2001 and 2002–2014 periods, past-month marijuana use remained more likely among middle-class whites than among middle-class minorities.

Hard drug use was more common among middle-class whites than among middle-class minorities in 1994, and past-month hard drug use followed the same basic patterns for both groups between 1994 and 1998 and also between 1999 and 2001. The more rapid decline in the past-month hard drug use prevalence rate among middle-class whites between 2002 and 2014, however, resulted in middle-class minorities being more likely to report past-month hard drug use than middle-class whites by 2014.

Trends in prescription painkiller misuse among the middle class follow the same racial trends as general prescription drug misuse. Prescription painkiller misuse was much more common among middle-class whites than middle-class minorities in 1994. The much larger increase in past-month prescription painkiller misuse between 1994 and 1998 among middle-class minorities and the continued increases in the prescription painkiller misuse prevalence rate across the 1999–2001 and 2002–2014 period occurred during a period in which the prescription painkiller misuse rate among middle-class whites declined precipitously. The result of these trends was that middle-class minorities were more likely than middle-class whites to report past-month prescription painkiller misuse in 2014.

With the exception of a spike in heroin use among middle-class minorities around 1999, middle-class heroin use prevalence rates were very low across the 1993–1998 and 1999–2001 periods. Between 2002 and 2014, however, the past-month heroin use rate among middle-class whites doubled, whereas the past-month heroin use rate among middle-class minorities declined during this same period. By 2014, heroin use was a much bigger problem among middle-class whites than among middle-class minorities.

The best conclusion that can be drawn about the racialized nature of the prescription drug misuse problem in the United States is that middle-class whites do indeed have a unique problem with prescription drug misuse. Compared with the drug use patterns of middle-class minorities in the United States, middle-class white Americans are disproportionately involved in prescription drug misuse than other forms of drug use. That data also reveal, however, that heroin is substantially more likely among middle-class whites than middle-class minorities, a trend that has grown rapidly in recent years.

The ultimate conclusion is that yes, the American middle-class, regardless of gender and social class, does have a marginally unique problem with prescription drug misuse than lower-income Americans. Although the American middle class misuses prescription medications at a lower rate than lower-income groups in the United States, compared with the income gap in other drugs, middle-class Americans are indeed overrepresented in the prescription drug misuse problem in the United States. Middle-class women and middle-class whites are also disproportionately represented in the population of prescription drug misusers compared with middle-class men and middle-class minorities. Prescription painkiller misuse, however, is an exception to the middle-class race gap in overall prescription drug misuse. Middle-class minorities misuse prescription painkillers at a higher rate than middle-class whites, and the middle-class race gap in prescription painkiller misuse is larger than for overall prescription drug misuse and is more in line with the middle-class race gap in the use of other drugs.

The most notable trend in middle-class drug abuse patterns described above, however, is the rapid increase in heroin use among middle-class women in the United States that occurred between 2002 and 2014. This rapid increase in heroin use among middle-class women was unmatched by increases in heroin use among any other demographic group addressed in this analysis and was accompanied by a noteworthy decrease in prescription painkiller misuse. Middle-class women have an emerging major problem with heroin use.

Is Prescription Drug Misuse a Disease of Despair?

A report published in 2015 in the *Proceedings of the National Academy of Sciences of the United States of America* by two Princeton University economists, Anne Case and Angus Deaton, revealed a striking discovery in death statistics in the United States from 1999 to 2013. The trend in the United States and all other industrialized nations over the past several decades had been substantial and sustained reductions in mortality rates for middle-age adults. Between 1970 and 2013, for example, mortality rates (i.e., the risk of death) for people in the United States between 45 and 54 years of age decreased by 44 percent, largely as a result of significant improvements in health care and behavioral changes. This report demonstrated that the United States and other industrialized nations continued to show declines in mortality rates for middle-age adults, with one notable exception—mortality rates for white Americans *increased* between 1999 and 2013. Specifically, the report determined that the increase in death rates among white middle-age Americans was concentrated among *non–college-educated whites.* Mortality rates decreased for middle-age college-educated white Americans, degree or not, during this period. The increase in mortality was due to increases in what the authors call "diseases of despair"—lung cancer, liver disease, suicides, and poisonings (mostly from prescription drugs). Of these causes of death, poisonings were responsible for the vast majority of the increase in mortality rates among noncollege white Americans.

Income inequality and economic instability became particularly pressing concerns for noncollege white Americans born into the baby boom generation. Anne Case and Angus Denton remark on the degree of desperation found among this population:

> Although the epidemic of pain, suicide, and drug overdoses preceded the financial crisis, ties to economic insecurity are possible. After the productivity slowdown in the early 1970s, and with widening income inequality, many of the baby-boom generation are the first to find, in midlife, that they will not be better off than were their parents. Growth in real median earnings has been slow for this group, especially those with only a high school education. However, the productivity slowdown is common to many rich countries, . . . yet none have had the same mortality experience. The United States has moved primarily to defined-contribution pension plans with associated stock market risk, whereas, in Europe, defined-benefit pensions are still the norm. Future financial insecurity may weigh more heavily on US workers, if they perceive stock market risk harder to manage than earnings risk, or if they have contributed inadequately to defined-contribution plans.[11]

In short, middle-age baby boomer noncollege white Americans have suffered from large-scale economic shifts in the United States, and it is possible that the insecurity and economic inequality among this group have created despair that has led to persistent problems with alcohol, tobacco, and drug use, including prescription drug misuse. Because the Centers for Disease Control and Prevention does not report death statistics by income, no analysis as to whether middle-class Americans were disproportionately impacted by the prescription drug *death* epidemic is possible. The death statistics on middle-age noncollege white Americans, however, is distressing and warrants a further investigation of prescription drug misuse as a disease of despair among this group.

Table 16 shows the drug use patterns of noncollege white Americans in the NSDUH, including various subgroups within this population, to determine if noncollege whites experienced noticeably different trends in prescription drug misuse from 1994 to 2014. The first column in the table includes all white Americans without any college education. In general, noncollege white Americans showed prescription drug misuse rates higher than the U.S. population as a whole across this period, but the increase in prescription drug misuse between 1999 and 2001 was three

Table 16. Past-Month Drug Use Patterns among Noncollege Whites, 1994–2014

	Noncollege White Males	Noncollege Whites	Noncollege Whites 35+	Noncollege White Males, <$20k, 18–24	U.S. Population Total
Prescription Drug Misuse					
% Change 1994–1998	18.6%	14.3%	208.3%	14.2%	55.1%
	(0.97%–1.15%)	(0.77%–0.88%)	(0.12%–0.37%)	(1.48%–1.69%)	(0.49%–0.76%)
% Change 1999–2001	74.6%	64.5%	91.7%	18.5%	20.7%
	(1.69%–2.95%)	(1.55%–2.55%)	(0.84%–1.61%)	(7.02%–8.32%)	(1.64%–1.98%)
% Change 2002–2014	–3.6%	–14.0%	–19.8%	–44.0%	–10.1%
	(3.02%–2.91%)	(2.93%–2.52%)	(1.97%–1.58%)	(8.35%–4.68%)	(2.58%–2.32%)
Marijuana Use					
% Change 1994–1998	40.1%	51.8%	177.4%	74.3%	37.9%
	(3.74%–5.24%)	(2.45%–3.72%)	(0.62%–1.72%)	(7.86%–13.70%)	(2.35%–4.00%)
% Change 1999–2001	23.7%	28.8%	56.6%	24.2%	14.2%
	(6.62%–8.19%)	(4.51%–5.81%)	(1.96%–3.07%)	(20.74%–25.76%)	(4.57%–5.22%)
% Change 2002–2014	43.9%	59.2%	112.4%	12.1%	38.1%
	(9.00%–12.95%)	(6.25%–9.95%)	(3.07%–6.52%)	(25.82%–28.95%)	(6.04%–8.34%)
Hard Drug Use					
% Change 1994–1998	44.9%	47.3%	–48.1%	155.7%	45.0%
	(0.89%–1.29%)	(0.55%–0.81%)	(0.27%–0.14%)	(2.55%–6.52%)	(0.60%–0.87%)
% Change 1999–2001	30.4%	20.2%	4.0%	101.6%	12.4%
	(1.48%–1.93%)	(1.14%–1.37%)	(0.50%–0.52%)	(4.25%–8.57%)	(1.13%–1.27%)
% Change 2002–2014	–20.3%	–12.6%	1.9%	–34.3%	–19.9%
	(1.72%–1.37%)	(1.19%–1.04%)	(0.53%–0.54%)	(5.51%–3.62%)	(1.46%–1.17%)

Prescription Painkiller Misuse					
% Change 1994–1998	65.3%	–36.7%	125.0%	inf.	80.0%
	(0.49%–0.81%)	(0.38%–0.60%)	(0.12%–0.27%)	(0.00%–0.50%)	(0.30%–0.54%)
% Change 1999–2001	87.1%	75.5%	94.1%	68.7%	28.8%
	(1.16%–2.17%)	(1.02%–1.79%)	(0.51%–0.99%)	(4.03%–6.80%)	(1.11%–1.43%)
% Change 2002–2014	6.0%	–4.2%	–2.7%	–47.4%	–13.7%
	(2.16%–2.29%)	(1.91%–1.83%)	(1.13%–1.10%)	(6.27%–3.30%)	(1.82–1.57%)
Heroin Use					
% Change 1994–1998	–100.0%	–95.0%	–100.0%	0.0%	–50.0%
	(0.44%–0.00%)	(0.20%–0.01%)	(0.27%–0.00%)	(0.00%–0.00%)	(0.08%–0.04%)
% Change 1999–2001	100.0%	700.0%	0.0%	16.1%	–16.7%
	(0.02%–.0.04%)	(0.01%–0.08%)	(0.00%–0.00%)	(0.31%–0.36%)	(0.06%–0.05%)
% Change 2002–2014	380.0%	400.0%	600.0%	–77.5%	142.9%
	(0.05%–0.24%)	(0.04%–0.20%)	(0.01%–0.07%)	(0.71%–0.16%)	(0.07%–0.17%)

Source: 1994–2014 NSDUH

times greater among this group than the U.S. population. Marijuana and hard drug use among noncollege white Americans were lower than the U.S. population across this period, and the changes in marijuana and hard drug use were generally the same as the U.S. population as a whole. Prescription painkiller abuse, however, was slightly more prevalent across the study period among noncollege whites than the U.S. population and, like prescription drug misuse, increased about three times faster from 1999 to 2001 than among the U.S. population as a whole. Heroin use among noncollege white Americans increased rapidly and emerged as a more significant issue among this group than in the United States as a whole after 1998.

The next three columns show drug use patterns for noncollege white males, noncollege whites above the age of 35 (includes the 45–54 age range analyzed in the study described above), and noncollege young (18–25), poor (<$20,000) white males. Noncollege white males showed drug use patterns very similar to the patterns among noncollege white Americans as a whole, with the exception that their past-month drug use rates are generally higher. The one notable exception is that although prescription drug misuse rates declined for noncollege white males from 2002 to 2014, albeit more slowly than noncollege whites and the U.S. population as a whole, prescription painkiller misuse rates increased for noncollege white males during this period. Drug use patterns among noncollege white middle-age Americans are also similar to the patterns shown by the entire group of noncollege white Americans, but the prevalence use rates among this group are generally lower for this group than for all noncollege whites in the United States. Prescription drug misuse, however, increased more rapidly among middle-age noncollege whites from 1999 to 2001 than among noncollege whites as a whole or noncollege white males during this period. In fact, the prescription drug misuse rate among middle-age noncollege whites increased almost five times faster from 1999 to 2001 than among the U.S. population as a whole. The group of middle-age noncollege whites also showed more rapid increases in prescription painkiller misuse across this same period.

The data show that noncollege white Americans were more strongly affected by the growing prescription drug misuse problem in the United States than any other demographic group. The most striking patterns of drug use, however, were shown among young, poor, noncollege white males. Changes in drug use over the period investigated are certainly noteworthy, especially the very substantial increases in hard drug use from 1994 to 2001 among this group, but more noteworthy are the overall percentages of this population who misused prescription drugs and used other drugs across the study period. An average of more than 10 percent of young, poor, noncollege white males, for instance, reported past-month prescription drug misuse between 2004 and 2011, and an average of more than 8 percent of this population reported past-month prescription painkiller abuse over the same period, 3 to 4 times the rates of prescription drug and prescription painkiller misuse rates among the U.S. population as a whole. Rates of past-month hard drug use ranged between 5 percent and 7 percent across most of the 20 years of data, compared with just over 1 percent past-month hard drug use rates for the U.S. population over this period. Past-month marijuana use rates were between 25 percent and 33 percent of the young, poor, noncollege white male population in the years between 2002 and 2014, rates that were 4 to 6 times higher than the United States as a whole. Nearly 1 percent of young, poor, noncollege white males reported past-month heroin use in 2013, nearly 10 times the past-month heroin use rate among the U.S. population in the same year.

To the degree that noncollege white Americans have experienced increases in social and economic despair over the past two decades, prescription drug misuse has followed. Noncollege white Americans did experience unique increases in prescription drug misuse, including prescription painkiller abuse, over the past 20 years. Middle-age noncollege white baby boomers experienced rapid increases in prescription drug misuse, especially between 1999 and 2001, but the absolute prevalence rates of drug use and prescription drug misuse remain lower than for the United States as a whole. The increased mortality rates among this population, however, are not necessarily accounted for in the prescription drug *misuse* or heroin use prevalence rates. The poisoning mortality increases from 1999 to 2013 among this group might be evidence of despair, but the despair was expressed in more deadly drug use patterns among a very small portion of the middle-age noncollege white population, not in the wide-scale misuse of prescription medications or heroin use.

Of all drug use patterns examined throughout this book, the population of young, poor, noncollege white males is most distressing. Compared to the U.S. drug use patterns as a whole, the population of young, poor, noncollege white males uses drugs in all forms, including the misuse of prescription drugs and prescription painkillers, at terrifyingly high rates. Middle-age noncollege white Americans are experiencing an increase in mortality rates during a time of steady and substantial declines in mortality rates for other Americans in the same age range and citizens of other

Western nations, and the increased mortality rates are largely due to a rapid increase in drug use poisonings. Clearly, intervention and prevention efforts are needed that address prescription drug misuse among this population. But the despair evidenced by remarkably higher rates of prescription drug misuse among young, poor, noncollege white males is striking and in desperate need of public attention.

CHAPTER FOUR

Policy Prescriptions

Prescription drug misuse is clearly a problem in the United States, particularly—as discussed in the previous chapter—the misuse of prescription opioid medications among young, poor, non–college-educated white Americans. Additionally, the stereotypical face of drug use in the United States has been fundamentally altered by the overrepresentation of females, rural residents, older people, whites, the middle class, and people with college educations in the drug use prevalence statistics. Most distressingly, the prescription drug misuse *death* epidemic is heavily concentrated among groups not typically associated with drug use, including whites, females, and rural residents. This changing face of drug use, including the exponentially increasing mortality associated with prescription drug misuse, has likely contributed to the current drug use paradigm that is dominated by prevention and rehabilitation. As highlighted throughout this book, drug treatment stands in stark contrast to the criminal justice approach to all prior drug scares. That said, prescription drug misuse prevention and rehabilitation does have a criminal justice element, mainly in the form of prescription drug monitoring programs (PDMPs), which are described in detail below. Operated and managed in part by law enforcement officials, PDMPs are still in line with epidemiological or public health approaches to the problem. Although arrest and incarceration of prescription drug misusers is part of PDMPs, the stated goal of these programs is to reduce the illegal diversion of prescription medication. Stated differently, PDMPs are designed to limit access to prescription medications that are often misused and hopefully reduce demand for illegal prescription drugs.

This chapter is devoted to describing and analyzing various programs designed to reduce prescription drug misuse as well as prescription drug overdose deaths. Prescription opioids are clearly the emphasis for most of these programs. The programs described below include PDMPs, medication-assisted treatment (MAT), and Narcan (the opioid overdose prevention medicine). The descriptions and analyses of the prescription drug misuse and death treatment and prevention programs, however, are complicated by the fact that all of these programs are created and managed by local and state authorities. To date, there has not been any federal policy in the United States to address the prescription drug misuse and death problem beyond the legislation that categorizes drugs and mandates prescriptions to obtain and possess the medications. Even drug treatment that is now offered through Medicaid, a health insurance program administered by the U.S. government, varies from state to state. Because of the vast variation in local and state approaches to addressing the prescription drug misuse problem, it is nearly impossible to identify what works to prevent and treat prescription drug misuse and overdose deaths. There are, however, some commonalities among the various programs that have shown some degree of success, which we describe throughout the chapter.

Prescription Drug Monitoring Programs

PDMPs are statewide electronic databases of specifically prescribed drugs.[1] PDMPs retain information on how prescribed drugs are dispensed within a particular state. The information that is retained in the PMDP may be accessed by authorized individuals or organizations based on state law.[2] In many situations, those eligible to access the information are prescribers, law enforcement officials, and licensing boards.

PDMPs are part of a larger tracking system that began at the turn of the 20th century. For instance, in 1914 New York state enacted a law requiring physicians to use a serialized duplicate form when prescribing certain drugs.[3] These duplicate forms were kept to monitor the amount and frequency of prescriptions. New York state was not alone. In fact, California began a program in 1939 using triplicate forms for specified narcotics.[4] This program would be modified in the 1970s and 1980s to include Schedule II narcotics and Schedule II nonnarcotics.[5] Research showed that these programs, while innovative, were not very effective. The research indicated that problems with physicians ordering and using the forms was not consistent, thus reducing the ability to prescribe the proper medication. PDMPs are an advance on these earlier programs.[6]

Unlike the previous programs in New York state and California, today all 50 states, the District of Columbia, and the two U.S. territories (Guam and Puerto Rico) administer PDMPs in various ways. The administration of PDMPs is not the only difference; in some states, for instance, the organization that administers the PDMP differs as well. Some states have the pharmacy board, the health department, a professional licensing agency, law enforcement agencies, substance abuse agencies, or consumer protection agencies administer the PDMP.[7] Typically, the administration of the PDMP happens by either pharmacy boards or health departments.[8]

While the administration of the PDMP varies, the legal statute that governs the PDMP also varies by states. In general, state laws determine the types of drugs (i.e., schedules of controlled substances) that the PDMP will monitor.[9] In addition, the legal statutes determine the information that the PDMP will include, the manner of submission, and the amount of time that is necessary to submit the information.

The legal statutes in each state also provide which entity will submit the information to the PDMP. Most states require retail pharmacies and dispensing physicians to submit the information to the PDMP.[10] Importantly, the submitted information is not solely for prescriptions occurring within a specified state. Many states have the authority to require prescribing out-of-state, mail-order, and Internet pharmacies to submit their data to the PDMP with respect to the prescribing of controlled substance to a resident of that state.[11] For example, if an individual from Kentucky receives a prescription for a monitored drug from an Internet pharmacy, the Internet pharmacy has to report the prescription to the Kentucky PDMP.

Importantly, PDMPs do not keep information on all controlled substances. For instance, medications that are dispensed at federally assisted drug treatment programs often do not report to PDMPs without consent from the individual.[12] At issue here is the privacy of the individual. Federally, privacy laws are strict about the amount of information that may be shared, especially if it identifies the individual as a drug abuser.

State laws not only monitor the drugs that are dispensed and indicate who has to provide the information but also provide who may access the information.[13] PDMPs may maintain a wealth of information, but not everyone has access to it. A large number of states provide that only pharmacists and practitioners have access to this information. To further complicate the reporting process, the term "practitioners" may be rather open. In some states, practitioners may include law enforcement, licensing and regulatory boards, state Medicaid programs, state medical examiners, and research organizations.[14] While these entities have the potential to access the information from the PDMP, state law outlines the procedures necessary to obtain the data.

States also vary in use of the data from the PDMP. Here, two terms are relevant: "reactive use" and "proactive use." First, the idea of reactive use is important to understand. Reactive use is when an entity has been contacted for a report.[15] In other words, the entity is reacting to an inquiry that has been made by a pharmacist or practitioner. For example, a pharmacist notices an unusual number of monitored substances being prescribed in a short amount of time to the same individual. The pharmacist contacts the PDMP for a report about this individual. With the report, the pharmacist may take several courses of action, including refusing to fill the prescription or forwarding the issue to the appropriate authorities. Second, proactive use of PDMPs is important as well. Proactive use occurs when an authorized entity uses the information from the PDMP to investigate cases or generate unsolicited reports. For instance, law enforcement may use the information from the PDMP to investigate a physician who has been making suspicious prescriptions. These two uses highlight the potential uses of PDMP information, but these uses are consistently undermined by the inability to share information with other states.

At this point, it is instructive to reinforce that PDMPs vary in every part of their structure (i.e., database and governing legal statutes). Historically, these differences have created a number of problems in sharing their data.[16] Many states, however, have overcome these issues and developed memorandums of understanding (MOUs) to share their data. The MOUs are predicated on policy and reciprocity agreements between the states.[17] The primary issue with sharing PDMP information across states is the reluctance of most states to share information that could hinder ongoing investigations. Table 17 presents a number of questions and considered issues that are often part of MOUs across states in sharing their information.[18] These issues are usually covered in most MOUs. Without covering these issues, the effectiveness of sharing the PDMP data is not very effective.

The effectiveness of the PDMP is determined by its use. In other words, pharmacists and physicians have to be compelled and comply with state law to report the prescription data to the program.[19] Each state has differing consequences for those not complying with their laws. The possible consequences for not reporting information to the PDMP ranges from disciplinary reports issued to hearings in front of licensing and regulatory boards to criminal justice sanctions.

Are PDMPs effective in reducing the misuse of prescription medications? After all, the prevalence of prescription drug abuse in the United States has been declining nationwide for approximately a decade, during which states initiated and escalated PDMPs. The overall effectiveness of

Table 17. Questions and Issues in Sharing PDMP Information

Questions	Issues
How will the information be reported?	Education (i.e., responsibility of providers, data integrity, training requirements)
How will the information be used?	Funding (i.e., costs of data sharing and costs of operation)
What are the guidelines on data retention?	Security and Access (i.e., authorized users, authentication, Internet access, confidentiality, privacy)
What are the states responsibilities in the event of a data breach?	Technology (i.e., data transfer and exchange, uniformity in standards, cost reduction, quality/error check)
Are the measures in place for conflict resolution?	
What re the consequences of potential data misuse?	

Source: L. N., Sacco, J. H. Duff, and A. K. Sarata, *Prescription Drug Monitoring Programs* (Congressional Research Service, Washington, DC, 2018).

PDMPs cannot be specifically determined because PDMPs are operated at the state level, and each state structures PDMPs differently. The following description of the effectiveness of some PDMPs is not meant to be exhaustive; rather, the review is meant to provide some information about how PDMPs operate. Table 18 provides a summation of PDMPs for four states (Kentucky, Ohio, West Virginia, and Florida). These states have some of the larger issues with the nonmedical misuse of prescription drugs and strong PDMPs.

PDMPs can only be effective when pharmacists and physicians provide the information. As noted above, the effectiveness of PDMPs is difficult to assess because of the administrative variety across states. This hampers researchers' abilities to be able to perform national-level studies on PDMP effectiveness. To clarify, the commonalities of objectives and administration across states are so disparate that the PDMPs do not provide a solid foundation for national-level studies.[20] While some will argue that the outcomes of the PDMPs are potentially the same and that this should be enough to warrant a national-level study, in reality the subtle nuances of administration and use of the PDMP may mask a national-level outcome.[21] Regardless, some research has taken place on individual states' PDMPs.

One way to examine information on PDMPs using research on states is to examine each of the studies and combine them into a research summary

Table 18. Select PDMPs

State	# of Pharmacies in State	# of Practitioners	Frequency of Data	Data Collection: Pharmacies	Data Collection: Dispensing Practitioners	Schedules Monitored	Allowed Requesters from PDMP	Legislation	Year Operational
Florida	5,019	84,161	Daily	Yes	Yes	II, III, IV, V	Prescribers, pharmacists, law enforcement, licensing boards. Others may also request but are not guaranteed.	FL Statute §§893.055 to .0551	2011
Kentucky	1,198	19,929	Daily	Yes	Yes	II, III, IV, V, and Nalbuphine (Schedule IV), Gabapentin (Schedule V)	Prescribers, pharmacists, law enforcement, licensing boards. Others may also request but are not guaranteed.	KY Rev Statute §218A.202; §§218A.240; 218A.245; 218A.172; 218A.390; 218A.391	1999
Ohio	2,478	57,182	Daily	Yes	Yes	II, III, IV, V, and Gabapentin (12-1-16), medical marijuana (9-8-16)	Prescribers, pharmacists, law enforcement, licensing boards. Others may also request but are not guaranteed.	OH Rev Code §§4729.75 to .86; 4729.99; 4725.092; 4723.487; 4715.302; 4729.162; 4730.53; 4731.055	2006
West Virginia	584	9,292	Daily	Yes	Yes	II, III, IV, V, and opioid antagonists, Gabapentin	Prescribers, pharmacists, law enforcement, licensing boards. Others may also request but are not guaranteed.	WV Code §§60A-9-1 to -7; 16-1-4	1995

Source: "State Profiles," Prescription Drug Monitoring Program Training and Technical Assistance Center, http://www.pdmpassist.org/content/state-profiles.

or synthesis. Worley produced this type of study. Worley's study summarizes all of the available published research on PDMP effectiveness.[22] The results indicated that PDMPs are effective in three areas. First, the research shows that PDMPs are effective in reducing doctor shopping. Doctor shopping is when an individual will visit multiple physicians to obtain a prescription or sizable quantities of the prescription. Second, the research shows that PDMPs are effective in changing prescribing behavior.[23] Specifically, physicians and pharmacists have become hesitant in prescribing monitored medications in their practices that may not be necessary. Third, the research shows that PDMPs are effective in reducing prescription drug misuse. Subsequent research has supported these results. In addition, in 2015 a group of Kentucky researchers showed that PDMPs are effective in closing non–physician-owned pain management facilities.[24] Other studies show that PDMPs are associated with a reduction in the rates of prescription opioid poisoning.[25]

Drug Treatment

PDMPs are designed to help reduce instances of the nonmedical use of prescription drugs through monitoring. Other mechanisms are influential in reducing misuse instances of the nonmedical use of prescription drugs. Drug treatment bears particular import in this area.

Before delving into drug treatment, it is instructive to understand what biological and psychological effects are produced by the misuse of prescription drugs. In the beginning of the prescription drug misuse process, the individual receives an initial euphoric event. The euphoric event may create cravings for additional euphoric events.[26] Research indicates that the continued (i.e., long-term) euphoric events create substantial changes in the individual's brain.[27] The brain changes that occur causes the individual to have other problems that include reduction in impulse control. With the reduction of impulse control, the continued misuse of prescription drugs is probable. The probability of this type of behavior increases when the individual encounters psychological stress, family problems, psychiatric illness, or social or environmental cues.[28] These issues threaten the chances for a reduction in misuse. Drug treatment is able to assist in this reduction.

Drug treatment can be defined in multiple ways. Here, we refer to drug treatment as multiple methods designed to assist individuals who misuse prescription drugs in reducing or stopping their compulsive seeking or use.[29] Within this definition, we view multiple methods as including medications and counseling. We also see the compulsive seeking or use as similar to addiction. Drug treatment is therefore important for reducing an individual's instances of the nonmedical misuse of prescription drugs.

Because the misuse of prescription drugs has varied effects on individuals, multiple forms of drug treatment are necessary. The inherent biological changes that are created in the misuse of prescription medications suggests that interpretation of life's issues may vary by individual.[30] In other words, individuals will have different cues that will create the necessity for different forms of drug treatment.[31] This means that drug treatment may take place in different settings, forms, and lengths of time.

Different forms and lengths of drug treatment are important. For instance, some may require behavioral therapies, while others may require the use of medications. Some individuals, however, may require the use of both behavioral therapies and medications. For many, drug treatment may last for different lengths of time. Given the open-ended nature of drug treatment, some principles of drug treatment are important. The National Institute of Drug Addiction provides a number of principles of effective drug treatment.[32] Table 19 provides the principles of effective drug treatment.

These principles indicate that important parts of drug treatment must be adhered to. In the context of the nonmedical use of prescription drugs, these principles are seen the most in MAT therapies.

MAT is a multipronged approach to substance use treatment.[33] MATs make use of medications and counseling and behavioral therapies to reduce instances of substance use. This approach is an attempt to provide a holistic, or whole-person, approach to substance use.

While MATs have shown promise for multiple types of substances, the approach often is used to treat opioid and prescription opioid addiction and use. In general, medications in MATs chemically treat a portion of the body. For instance, medications used in MATs work to block the euphoric effects of opioids and reduce the psychological cravings.[34] MATs use medications to provide normality in an individual's body without the negative effects (i.e., withdrawal) of the abused drug.[35] MATs, however, do not just rely on medication to treat the effects of substance use.

MATs also make use of counseling and behavioral therapy. Counseling and behavioral therapy may vary depending on the individuals' needs. In general, counseling involves two formats (i.e., group and individual sessions). Group sessions involve small groups of individuals who have similar afflictions. Counselors usually attend these sessions and provide an opportunity for everyone to share their feelings and behaviors revolving around their substance misuse.[36]

Individual sessions tend to be more intense, with the individual working one-on-one with the counselor or therapist. These sessions work to

Table 19. Principles of Effective Drug Treatment

Misuse is complex and influence bran functioning.
Proper treatment differs for everyone.
Immediacy of drug treatment is paramount for success.
Effective drug treatment seeks to focus on multiple needs of the individual, not just misuse.
Staying in treatment for the proper amount of time is critical.
Behavioral therapies are essential.
Medications are an important element of drug treatment.
Treatment plans must be dynamic to change as the individual's needs change.
Misuse usually co-occurs with mental disorders, so both need to be treated.
Medical detoxification is only the first stage of addiction treatment and by itself does little to change long-term drug abuse.
Treatment does not need to voluntary to be effective.
Treatment must be monitored continuously.
Treatment programs must test for the presence of other diseases (e.g., HIV, AIDS, hepatitis).

Source: U.S. Department of Health and Human Services, Substance Abuse and Mental Health Services Administration, *Results from the 2016 National Survey on Drug Use and Health: Summary of National Findings*, July 2018, https://www.samhsa.gov/data/sites/default/files/NSDUH-FFRI-2016/NDSUH-FFR1-2016.htm.

arrive at the etiology and continuation of the substance misuse. In these sessions, counselors attempt to assist individuals' with emotional and behavioral techniques that will improve their opportunities for successfully reducing instances of nonmedical prescription drug misuse.[37]

An overlooked part of MATs is the human capital portion. MAT participation requires vocational and educational training. As often occurs, individuals who misuse substances are often without an education or a vocation.[38] MAT provides an opportunity to become educated, train, or retrain for a different vocation. These professionals provide a variety of therapies. Table 20 provides the types of therapies that counselors are able to provide.

Here we focus on three forms of MAT. The first is cognitive-behavioral therapy (CBT), which attempts to help individuals replace faulty thinking that leads to antisocial behavior or "negative emotions."[39] In other words, interventions in CBT focus on changing the individual's thoughts. Changing the thoughts results in changing the individual's behavior or emotional state.

Table 20. Types of MAT Therapies

Cognitive-behavioral therapy (CBT) trains the individual to do two things. First, the therapy trains individuals to recognize their patterns of negative thinking or behaviors. Second, the therapy trains individuals or provides techniques to stop the patterns of negative thinking or behaviors. Tangibly, this type of therapy helps individuals become aware of stressors, situations, and feelings that often lead to substance misuse.
Contingency management therapy (CMT) provides incentives to reinforce positive behaviors. Positive behaviors that receive reinforcement include abstinence from substance misuse.
Motivational enhancement therapy (MET) revolves around planning. Individuals taking part in this type of therapy work to build motivation and commit specific plans to engage in treatment and therapy.
Twelve-step facilitation therapy uses the tactics in popular 12-step programs such as Alcoholics Anonymous and Narcotics Anonymous.

Source: E. Dyb, "Housing First or No Housing? Housing and Homelessness at the End of the Alcohol and Drug Treatment," *International Journal on Drug Policy* 36 (2016): 76–84.

Beck assumes that antisocial behavior and disturbed mood or emotions are the result of improper behaviors, know as automatic thoughts.[40] The individual, when in a situation, may react in a manner not consistent with reality but instead with a distorted point of view.[41] The purpose of CBT is to make the individual aware of the distortion and help the individual use techniques to restructure the cognition. The behavioral portion of the therapy trains the individual in how to replace the undesirable behavior. The focus is not on uncovering the motivations behind the behavior but instead is on changing the behavior.

CBT is a combination of these two therapies. A counselor helps an individual identify both the thoughts and behaviors that are causing issues and helps the individual change those thoughts in order to readjust the behavior. CBT is a general form of therapy. In other words, this may be applied to all genres of life, and CBT has been applied to several forms of disorders (i.e., mental disorders, mood disorders, personality disorders, and substance abuse).[42] While it is general in nature, the therapy should not be used with everyone struggling with drug-related and other disorders. For instance, those individuals who are more interested in the past rather than overcoming a disorder probably should not use CBT. In addition, individuals who have cognitive disorders (e.g., traumatic brain injury) are probably not good candidates for CBT.

CBT utilizes a number of techniques, a few of which are as follows:

1. Behavioral homework assignments: A counselor provides an individual with homework. The homework may include experiments that help the individual see differences in behavior during situations.
2. Cognitive rehearsal: The individual is asked to imagine difficult situations, and the counselor is able to assist in a step-by-step process of facing the situation. The individual then rehearses the steps mentally.
3. Journal: The individual keeps a journal to help in being aware of her or his thoughts, feelings, or actions.
4. Modeling: The individual and the therapist engage in role-playing activities.
5. Conditioning: The individual uses reinforcement to encourage a particular behavior.
6. Systematic desensitization: The individual imagines a situation that he or she fears, and the counselor helps the individual relax and cope with the fear reaction.
7. Validity testing: The therapist asks the individual to provide evidence that the thoughts the individual is producing are true.[43]

The collaborative nature of CBT dictates that the individual and the counselor spend time working to gain rapport and a general understanding of how the therapy works. When this is accomplished, the environment for therapy is action oriented. The action orientation gives the individual a sense of empowerment and an active role. The individual becomes less dependent on the counselor. Beck argues that some of the therapy practices do not last very long (approximately 16 weeks).

In addition to CBT, contingency motivation therapy is another option. This form of therapy is based on motivation. Motivation is an important factor for successful recovery from substance use disorders.[44] Deci and Ryan provide two major categories of motivation.[45] Intrinsic motivation is based on an individual producing a behavior because it brings inherent satisfaction. Extrinsic motivation is apparent when individuals produce a behavior because they are expecting or promised some form of a reward. Contingency management is an important form of treatment because it uses external motivation to promote sustained recovery. In other words, contingency management interventions rely on the principles from operant conditioning. Operant conditioning emphasizes that a reward for a particular behavior is likely to encourage the repetition of that behavior. In this form of intervention, individuals are rewarded for abstinence or reduced use.[46] Rewards in this type of intervention are vouchers, clinical privileges, money, or other desirable items. The rewards provide positive reinforcement. The difference between contingency management and other psychological forms of intervention is that they do not emphasize the role of introspection or flaws in one's cognition (i.e., CBT). Rather, the emphasis is on reinforcement mechanisms. To date, researchers show that contingency management approaches are successful. Ainscough, McNeill, Strang, Calder, and Brose produced a meta-analysis of contingency management interventions from 22 studies to show that the approach is efficacious for reducing most drug use during treatment for opioids.[47] While this is an important finding, central to treatment is the long-term effect. In other words, the length that the individual will continue a behavior is likely to be contingent on a series of rewards. However, when the rewards cease, the likelihood of the continued behavior is likely to cease as well. Sayegh, Huey, Zara, and Jhaveri produced a meta-analysis of 84 studies showing that contingency management interventions provide limited effects on drug use during three- to six-month follow-ups.[48] These results are not to say that contingency management interventions are not successful or useful. To encourage continued recovery, these interventions need to make sure that their type of reward is something that may be able to be sustained after treatment has ceased.

These forms of therapy can be administered in multiple settings.[49] These settings may include hospitals and remote clinics that provide inpatient and residential treatment programs. Two types of inpatient and residential settings are possible. First, longer-term residential treatment may take place from 6 months to 12 months. While this type of treatment is uncommon, these settings provide a substantial amount of structure. The high level of structure allows the individual to embrace the MAT format. Second, short-term residential treatment primarily emphasizes detoxification (i.e., withdrawal). Short-term residential treatment provides intensive treatment within a community (i.e., clinic) setting.

In addition, MAT administration can occur in offices and is often on an intensive outpatient basis. These programs tend to have regular and intense meetings multiple times a week. The regular and intense sessions often occur initially, but less frequent meetings assist in sustaining individuals' recovery thereafter. Office settings for treatment are relevant because the individuals are often involved with a criminal issue. For those dealing with a concurrent criminal issue, administration of MAT can occur in correctional facilities, which greatly increases the populations whom MATs reach.

At this point, the discussion has been about general MATs. Specifically, opioid treatment programs (OTPs) are the emphasis of most MATs and treat prescription opioid misuse in addition to the use of heroin and other illicit opioids. OTPs' intentions are designed to improve the lives of the individuals who participate in them. This includes providing a range of services, including reducing, eliminating, or preventing the use of illicit drugs as well as potential criminal activity and the spread of infectious disease. Addressing these issues is consistent with the general structure of MATs.

MATs and OTPs use specific medications in their processes. Some popular medications are methadone and naloxone. Methadone is a medication used to help individuals who are addicted to opioids, including prescription opioids. This medication is a safe and effective way to help them recover from their substance misuse. Importantly, methadone works best as part of a comprehensive MAT. Methadone works by changing individuals' biology. One way this works is by changing their brain system to reduce cravings. Another way is by changing the individual's nervous system. With these changes, the individual responds to pain differently.[50] Methadone has the desirable properties to reduce painful symptoms of withdrawal. Further, methadone provides a euphoria block for opioids.

Methadone can be ingested in pill, liquid, or wafer form. The drug must be taken one time per day. A typical dosage of methadone lasts about four to eight hours. The power of methadone requires individuals to begin ingestion of the drug under the supervision of a physician.[51] After individual become stable in their treatment, they may be able to take their dosage of methadone at home between clinic visits. Methadone has to be part of a larger MAT plan for individuals, and the period of time in this treatment program will vary from person to person (i.e., months to years).

Methadone, however, is also dangerous. First, methadone can be addictive. This is the primary reason that individuals must begin their ingestion of the drug under the supervision of a physician. This helps to ensure that the proper dosage is taken. The addiction to methadone usually occurs when the individual takes the medication outside of the supervision of a physician. Second, methadone should never be shared with anyone because it is tailored to the individual who is receiving the medication. Third, methadone will interact with other medications. This means that individuals need to provide a complete history of the medications they are taking. A complete history may help the individual avoid larger problems (i.e., potential heart conditions). Further, the active ingredients of methadone tend to linger in the individuals' body. This is important to understand so that the individual does not unintentionally overdose.[52]

Methadone is serious medication with a number of side effects. Table 21 presents the potential side effects of methadone.

Table 21. Side Effects of Methadone

1. Difficulty breathing or shallow breathing.
2. Feeling light headed or faint.
3. Hives or rash.
4. Swelling of the face, lips, tongue, or throat.
5. Chest pains.
6. Fast or pounding heartbeat.
7. Hallucinations or confusion.

Source: B. K. Zedler et al., "Buprenorphine Compared with Methadone to Treat Pregnant Women with Opioid Use Disorder: A Systematic Review and Meta-analysis of Safety in the Mother, Fetus and Child," *Addiction* 111 (2016): 2131–2133.

Health Insurance, Medicaid, and the Affordable Care Act

While methadone and counseling comprise MAT, it is important to understand how these types of treatment are financed. Medicaid is a joint federal and state program that assists with medical costs. The Medicaid program helps individuals with limited income and resources. Medicaid also provides coverage for benefits not present in Medicare (e.g., nursing home care and personal care). For our purposes in this book, one of the more recent benefits of Medicaid is addiction treatment. Addiction coverage emerged in Medicaid because addiction has not historically been covered using private insurance. Research shows that more than 70 percent of addiction treatment financing comes from the government, with less than 15 percent of addiction financing comes from private insurance.[53] It is instructive to consider that some select Medicaid and private insurance plans focus on addiction but not on substance use disorders—the precursor to addiction.

Health care resources are limited, so focusing on those with the most serious need may be reasonable. This unfortunately creates a bifurcated system (i.e., a specialty system for those with addiction and those without addiction). The bifurcation effects the way the public and the medical community view addiction and the means to treat it. This is apparent when comparing addiction to other illnesses. McCellan and Woodworth compare addiction to diabetes.[54] Specifically, if insurance companies merely focused on those who are diabetic, this would eliminate prevention and early intervention efforts (i.e., prediabetes). Similarly, by focusing only on addiction, insurance programs would be ignoring the prevention and early intervention capabilities of medical professionals who address substance use disorders before such they develop into addictions.

Only treating diabetes once it is officially diagnosed, rather than treating the early indicators and preventing further development of the disease, creates complications related to external markets, labeling, and reductions in patient populations. For example, only treating officially diagnosed diabetes creates and enriches external markets, including groups or individuals who create screening or measurement instruments for diabetes.[55] These screening and measurement instruments will become the focus, because they will be able to identify diabetic individuals. This identification is likely to result in several different definition of diabetes, including prediabetes. The same issues occur with addiction. Specifically, screens and measurement instruments are built to better refine the definitions of substance use disorders and addiction.[56]

With the definition of the term "diabetes" under debate, some individuals will bear the label of diabetic just as many bear the label of addict. When thinking of a diabetic, these individuals will undergo psychological and sociological stigmatization. Overt shunning of individuals in a community may not occur, but as with addicts, shunning in the insurance community will occur.[57] Coverage will be more expensive for the diabetic as for the addict, and obtaining coverage may not occur at all. For diabetic individuals, the coverage will be difficult to obtain. In the United States employers are the primary health insurance provider, which means that individual employers determine the coverage for diabetes. The same applies to addiction. An employer would probably make the prudent decision to not offer health care that insures diabetes, as that coverage is more expensive for employers to provide.[58] The same applies to addiction. The cost of insurance that covers specialty care is prohibitive to many employers. Because private employer-sponsored health insurance that covers specialty care, including diabetes and addiction, is very expensive, prediabetic and substance use disorder intervention and treatment is not covered by many health insurance plans.

The comparison of diabetes and addiction provides an illustration of how insurance decisions may promote a perceptual change about an illness and influence how public and medical profession understand an illness. Further, this comparison provides an illustration of how those with diabetes may become part of a bifurcated system (i.e., a nondiabetic system and one for specialty care for those with diabetes). The general thought is that a separate specialty system for those with addiction and those without addiction exists.[59] In addition, the bifurcation is problematic because the precursor to addiction—substance abuse disorders—is not included.

Table 22. Key Issues from the Affordable Care Act

Require all Americans to purchase health care insurance.	Increases the number of insured individuals.
Enlarge the focus of the Centers for Medicare and Medicaid Services (CMS).	Allows this organization to do the following: (1) expand health care eligibility and (2) design health care provisions to reduce the variation in coverage financing.
Invest in prevention via financial incentives.	Abolish copays for patients and not require matching funds for states for prevention interventions.
Redesign chronic disease management.	Requires a team-based proactive approach to treat chronic illnesses.
Require health insurance plans and health care to include substance use disorders.	Substance use disorders will be treated as an essential service.

Source: A. T. McCellan and A. M. Woodworth, "The Affordable Care Act and Treatment for 'Substance Use Disorders': Implications of Ending Segregated Behavioral Healthcare," *Journal of Substance Abuse Treatment* 46 (2014): 541–545.

For many, addiction may be preventable. Early detection and intervention is necessary. However, most private insurance coverage does not provide for early intervention, nor did Medicaid—at least until Medicaid coverage expanded as part of the Affordable Care Act (ACA).[60]

The ACA is a wide-ranging change in health care coverage for low-income Americans. The changes in health care coverage are an attempt to reduce double-digit rate increases. Within the ACA, five major provisions, listed in Table 22, changed health care and the health care industry in the United States.

The adoption of the ACA led to the implementation of three key pieces of the legislation.[61] First, private insurance companies had to halt the practice of denying coverage to individuals with preexisting chronic illnesses (e.g., addiction). Second, employment changes did not result in the end of health care coverage, as individuals would be able to retain their health care insurance when changing employment. Third, families would be able to maintain coverage on their children through the age of 26. While the implementation of these three key pieces of the legislation are important, a large effect would be felt in the area of substance use disorders. Specifically, the ACA provided coverage for new populations who would not have otherwise had access to health insurance, including people who misuse prescription drugs, and the treatment available for drug users did not have to be based on addiction—substance use disorders (preaddiction) for prescription drug misuse or other forms of drug use became available with the ACA. Preaddiction is the precursor of addiction and occurs when an individual is exhibiting early signs and behaviors of addiction. Preaddiction will create a separate set of industries, including screening and measurement instruments that are sensitive enough to indicate a substance use disorder.

Another area that the ACA has influenced in the context of substance use disorders is the location of care. The increase in the amount of individuals who are available for care dictates changes in the type and location of care.[62] For instance, individuals with substance use disorder tendencies increased after the ACA's implementation. The large number of eligible individuals with substance use disorders pushed the specialty care treatment system. Some reports indicate that substance use disorders—including the nonmedical misuse of prescription drugs—impacts the lives of millions. The type of care has changed as well. For instance, rather than this type of treatment being left to counselors, primary care physicians are administering the treatment. This places a larger burden on primary care physicians to learn more about substance use disorders. PDMPs partly meet these educational needs. Overall, these changes have led to more questions than answers.

At the time of this writing, the ACA has come under attack politically. The attacks have led to repealing portions of the ACA. Even though pieces of the ACA have been repealed, a large number of states continue to use the expansions that it brought. The Henry Kaiser Foundation indicates as of July 2018 that 33 states have adopted the expansion of Medicaid, 14 states did not adopt the expansion of Medicaid, and 3 states are considering their adoption of expansion of Medicaid. Table 23 presents the specific states that continue the expansion.[63]

Naloxone (Narcan)

Naloxone is a medication as well. This medication is not designed to assist with addiction. Naloxone is designed to prevent overdoses of opioids, including prescription opioids.[64] Naloxone directly blocks the opioid receptor site in the brain. This reverses the toxic effects of opioids, and these qualities dictate that naloxone be administered when the individual shows signs of an overdose. The administration of naloxone may take place in several different ways (e.g., intranasal spray, intramuscular, under the skin, and intravenous injection).[65] Anyone can be trained to administer naloxone. Further, naloxone is safe for administration to pregnant women but only in limited doses and under the supervision of a physician.

Table 23. Medicaid Expansion by State

Adopted Expansion of Medicaid	Did Not Adopt Expansion of Medicaid	Considering Adopting Expansion of Medicaid
Alaska	Alabama	Idaho
Arizona	Florida	Nebraska
Arkansas	Georgia	Utah
California	Kansas	
Colorado	Mississippi	
Connecticut	Missouri	
Delaware	North Carolina	
District of Columbia	Oklahoma	
Hawaii	South Carolina	
Illinois	South Dakota	
Indiana	Tennessee	
Iowa	Texas	
Kentucky	Wisconsin	
Louisiana	Wyoming	
Maine		
Maryland		
Massachusetts		
Michigan		
Minnesota		
Montana		
Nevada		
New Hampshire		
New Jersey		
New Mexico		
New York		
North Dakota		
Ohio		
Oregon		
Pennsylvania		
Rhode Island		
Vermont		
Virginia		
Washington		
West Virginia		

Table 24. Withdrawal Symptoms of Naloxone

1. Feeling nervous, restless, or irritable.
2. Body aches.
3. Dizziness or weakness.
4. Diarrhea, stomach pain, or nausea.
5. Fever, chills, or goose bumps.
6. Sneezing or runny nose.

Source: D. Kerr, P. Dietze, and A. M. Kelly, "Intranasal Naloxone for the Treatment of Suspected Heroin Overdose," *Addiction* 103 (2008): 379–386.

Naloxone can also be prescribed. Coming from a physician, naloxone may be prescribed to individuals who are taking part in a MAT. Further, a physician may prescribe naloxone to an individual who is considered to be at risk for opioid overdose.[66] A number of criteria are necessary for an individual to be considered at risk for opioid overdose: taking high doses of opioids for long-term management of chronic pain, receiving rotating opioid medication regimens, having been recently discharged from emergency medical care for opioid poisoning or intoxication, taking certain extended-release or long-acting opioid medications, and completing detoxification.[67] Naloxone is not without danger. The medication does have a number of side effects and may create symptoms of withdrawal. The side effects are hives or swelling in the face, lips, or throat. Table 24 presents the symptoms of withdrawal using naloxone.

At the time of this writing, research on naloxone is limited. Cash, Kinsman, Crow, Rivard, Faul, and Panchal show that naloxone has been used rather extensively. Their study used data from the National Emergency Medical Services Information System. Cash et al. compare naloxone administrations from 2012 to 2016 opioid overdose mortality rates. Their results indicate that naloxone administration increased 75.1 percent, from 573.6 to 1004.4 administrations per 100,000 emergency medical service events. These administrations mirror the 79.7 percent increase in opioid overdose mortality from 7.4 deaths per 100,000 persons to 13.3.[68] Further, their research shows a bimodal age distribution of patients receiving naloxone. Cash et al. show a bimodal age distribution indicating that individuals between the ages of 25–34 and 45–54 are most likely to be given naloxone.

Conclusion

In this chapter we explored the role of PDMPs, drug treatment, and treatment for overdoses. PDMPs are relatively effective in reducing instances of the nonmedical use of prescription drugs. With all 50 states using PDMPs, their role is vital to succeeding in reducing instances of the nonmedical use of prescription drugs. Because of the variations and lack of communication between state PDMPs, however, firm conclusions about the degree of effectiveness in reducing prescription drug misuse are not possible. If the United States implements a comprehensive, standardized national PDMP strategy, stronger evidence as to how effective PDMPs are in reducing prescription drug misuse will be available. Beyond PDMPs, different forms of therapy are relevant to reducing the prescription drug misuse crisis in the United States. Specifically, CBT and contingency management therapy seem to have particular import for assisting those in recovery. Additionally, insurance changes associated with the ACA have expanded access to drug treatment, including prescription drug misuse, by covering a wider population and allowing treatment for preaddiction substance use disorders. Research on the effectiveness of expanded Medicaid coverage in reducing prescription drug misuse is forthcoming at the time of this writing, but if research shows positive effects of Medicaid expansion in reducing prescription drug misuse, other states should consider expanding Medicaid coverage and drug treatment access. Finally, naloxone has relevance when it comes to an overdose.

CHAPTER FIVE

Death and Destruction, Hope and Resilience

The stories of prescription drug misuse are distressing, the headlines are terrifying, and the future appears bleak. Prescription drug misuse appears to be destroying the United States, bringing death and destruction to countless individual lives and communities. Unlike prior drug crises in the United States, the prescription drug misuse crisis is unique because the substances that are seemingly destroying our communities are not only entirely legal in most situations but are also used legitimately to treat medical conditions ranging from mild anxiety to severe pain, with misuse often beginning with a medical prescription. How can medications that have improved the quality of life for so many Americans cause so much despair and destruction? Indeed, it is the perception that prescription medications are safe that drives many people to misuse them, often as an alternative to other seemingly more dangerous street drugs. The apparent "safety" of prescription drugs, however, stands in stark contrast to the prescription drug misuse death statistics.

In contrast to the media and political narrative being promoted about the prescription drug misuse crisis in the United States, the data show that prescription drug *misuse* rates are not entirely distressing. The fact is that past-month prescription drug misuse rates are relatively low—the 2014 National Survey on Drug Use and Health (NSDUH) showed that only 2.3 percent of people in the United States reported having misused any prescription medication in the past month. Further, the percentage of the U.S. population who reported past-month prescription drug misuse declined by 10.1 percent from 2002 to 2014. In contrast, the past-month marijuana use rate was 8.3 percent in 2014, and past-month marijuana use rates increased by 38.1 percent from 2002 to 2014. Prescription drug misuse is considerably less likely than marijuana use and has been decreasing in recent years during a period in which marijuana use has been skyrocketing in the United States. Compared to marijuana use, prescription drug misuse is therefore a relatively minor problem in the United States. The relatively low percentage of the U.S. population who misuse prescription drugs and the decreasing prescription drug misuse prevalence rates in recent years are glimmers of hope among the barrage of troubling headlines.

On the other hand, prescription drug misuse remains twice as likely as hard drug use in the United States. Prescription drug misuse became more prevalent than hard drug use in the mid-1990s, and the prevalence gap has widened in the years thereafter. Further, prescription drug misuse declined more slowly than hard drug use in the period between 2002 and 2014, and our data showed that prescription drug misuse did attract new and unique drug users over the past 20 years. Compared with hard drug use, prescription drug misuse is therefore a reason for concern. Even with the comparison to hard drug use, however, it cannot be ignored that prescription drug misuse afflicts a very small percentage of the U.S. population.

Despite the rarity of prescription drug misuse in the United States and recent declines in the prevalence of prescription drug misuse that clearly do not rise to the level of an epidemic from any official definition of the term, there are two glaring issues with the prescription drug misuse crisis in the United States that do justify significant and substantial public attention. The first pressing issue is that prescription drug misuse represents a change in the face of drug use in the United States, by which we mean that prescription drug misuse has infiltrated populations that have not traditionally been implicated in prior drug crises in the United States. Note, however, that prescription drug misuse is *not predominantly* a white, middle-class, female, college-educated, and/or rural problem. Rather, prescription drug use is a *more* white, middle-class, female, college-educated, and/or rural problem than marijuana or hard drug use. The changing drug use demographics associated with prescription drug misuse is essential to understanding the different public reactions to the prescription drug misuse problem and prior drug use problems in the United States, including the harsh criminal justice reaction to the crack problem in late 1980s and early 1990s. Illicit drug users are perceived as being different from "regular Americans"—immoral and dangerous—and that perception of immorality influences political and public reactions.

Prescription drug misusers, however, are perceived to be "normal Americans" who, through no fault of their own, became addicted to prescription medications, a perception that is reflected in the more lenient public and political reactions to the problem.

To better understand why the media and politicians have focused so heavily on the prescription drug misuse crisis and portrayed the prescription drug misuse problem as a public health crisis rather than a criminal justice issue, we turn to a very important research article on school shootings written by Charles E. Menifield and colleagues in the aftermath of several high-profile school shootings.[1] A reasonable question is *what do school shooting have to do with a drug use problem in the United States*? The answer to that question is quite simple: *unexpected* problems are more newsworthy and more warranting of sympathy than *expected* problems.

The locations and stories behind tragic school shootings have become part of the cultural lexicon in the United States. All Americans are familiar with the high-profile shooting events at Columbine, Sandy Hook, and, more recently, Parkland. Many Americans also know the stories behind shootings in Paducah, Kentucky; Jonesboro, Arkansas; Pearl, Mississippi; and, more recently, Marshall County, Kentucky. All of these shootings received considerable media and political attention. Television, print, radio, and Internet media organizations provided around-the-clock coverage of these events for days, weeks, and even years after the horrific events occurred. Because of the intense media coverage of these school shootings, these schools and stories have become the symbols of school violence across the United States. Focusing only on print media, Menifield and colleagues, however, pose the question, "Do the newspaper media present misleading views of school violence?"[2] After all, the highest-profile school shooting all occurred in rural areas, but earlier research concluded that 90 percent of all school shootings occur in urban schools.[3] Further, President Bill Clinton's task force on school violence, formed in reaction to several high-profile (rural) school shootings in the mid-1990s, found that "schools in cities were at least twice as likely to report serious violent crime as those in towns and rural locations."[4] If serious violence is mainly an urban problem, why do the media and politicians focus so heavily on the school shootings that occur in rural areas?

To answer this question and better understand the public's reaction to the prescription drug misuse problem in the United States, we need to understand the goals and role of the media in shaping how Americans think and feel about specific issues. Media has a powerful influence in shaping how people view and evaluate issues. One way the media is able to influence how consumers perceive a specific issue is through agenda setting. Because media, especially news media, cannot cover every story that occurs in a society, media has to select which stories to feature or address. Therefore, a media organization's decision to cover certain stories but ignore other stories tells consumers which stories are most important. By drawing attention to problems that need to be addressed and not giving attention to other stories that a media organization deems less important, the media functions as a filter for consumers. Research by Iyengar and Kinder on television news found support for this media function: "By attending to some problems and ignoring others, television news shapes the American public's political priorities."[5] Media therefore shows the American public which issues are most important and in need of public and political attention by choosing which stories to feature.

Priming is closely related to agenda setting. By directing the American public to be concerned about selected issues, media is also conditioning the American public to hold their elected officials accountable for their actions and solve the particular problem. In other words, Americans judge their elected officials on their success or failures in addressing the problems presented in the media. Relatively new societal problems, such as prescription drug misuse and school shootings, are particularly sensitive to the process of media priming—as the American public forms opinions about these new issues, the priming effect is more powerful than for more long-standing problems.

Beyond media outlets selecting topics to present to the public and priming the population to hold elective officials accountable on those selected problems, the media also decides how to present a topic. The way that media frames a particular issue has a powerful effect on how the population understands and evaluates that issue. With crime, for example, the media can frame a given crime problem as being caused by individual factors such as immorality, as the result of social issues such as poverty, or as a problem caused by a weak criminal justice system. Stated differently, "the thematic news frame places political issues and events in some general context."[6] The way media outlets frame an issue can have a dramatic impact on how consumers evaluate and understand the issues presented.

Because news media exists primarily to sell advertising and therefore generate profits, media outlets need to attract viewers, readers, and listeners. Decisions as to which stories to present to consumers are therefore made with specific intention to draw consumer attention to the stories. With the media coverage of school shootings, Menifield and associates show that newspapers were much more likely to cover rural school shootings than urban school shootings. Further, when newspapers presented rural school shootings, there were clear attempts to connect with the readers' emotional reactions to the story with multiple glaring pictures from the event and detailed stories of the victims. Rural school shootings were also much more likely to be presented on the front page of newspapers and to include significantly more words than urban school shootings. Finally, newspaper stories of rural school shootings gave considerable attention to understanding the motivations of the shooters, including intensive reporting on the family and school backgrounds of each school shooter. In contrast, newspaper coverage of urban school shootings tends to be very short, based mainly on the facts of the incident; to include very few (if any) pictures from the event; and to only mention the shooter in terms of the criminal justice process.

Newspapers therefore give more attention to rural school shootings (agenda setting), which primes the readers to hold elected officials accountable for their actions in addressing the problem of school shootings (priming) and frames the school shooting problem as an issue rooted in family and school problems (framing). On the other hand, newspaper coverage of urban school shootings is quite rare (agenda setting), which limits the public's demands of political officials to address urban school shootings (priming). When newspapers cover urban school shootings, the stories are short and to the point and do not attempt to explain the shooters' motivations, focusing almost exclusively on the criminal justice punishments associated with the shooting (framing). The result is that the American public views rural school shootings as a major problem that needs to be addressed by government officials, as the problem of rural school shootings is viewed as being caused by social problems, whereas urban school shootings are not an issue that needs attention from public officials and can be solved by criminal justice punishments.

The explanation provided by Menifield and associates for the disparate agenda setting, priming, and framing of school shootings based on whether the shootings occurred in rural or urban areas is quite simple—urban violence is expected, rural violence is not. Drawing from the work of Daniel Patrick Moynihan, it appears that our society has "defin[ed] deviancy down" for violence in urban areas—our culture is no longer shocked or outraged by urban violence, including shootings that occur in urban schools.[7] In contrast, violence in rural areas is still shocking and elicits outage in our culture simply because rural violence is seen as being rare. Menifield and associates summarize their findings with the following statement:

> It is clear that American newspapers treat urban and rural school crime differently. Apparently, the sheer amount of crime in urban schools (and urban areas) has desensitized the public and the media to it and thereby

> increased their tolerance of it. As a result, urban school violence simply is not new, and therefore it is not news. The grotesque happens so often it is no longer grotesque. . . . On the other hand, the rural incidents were new, they were uncommon and unexpected, and they *were* grotesque, so they, therefore, shocked both the public and the media and got their attention.[8]

Much in the same way that rural school shootings received more significant and prominent newspaper coverage than urban school shootings simply due to shock and dismay that rural violence continues to occur in our culture when rural violence is seen as being uncommon, prescription drug misuse is likely newsworthy only when it afflicts unexpected populations. Americans have come to expect drug use in urban areas and among males, poor people, racial and ethnic minorities, those who are poorly educated, and the young. In Moynihan's terms, Americans have defined drug use down among these specific populations. Additionally, attributions of blame for drug use among the groups that are *expected* to use drugs fall on the individual drug users themselves, and solutions are therefore based in criminal justice punishments. When drug use is perceived to be more common in rural areas and among females, wealthier people, whites, those with college educations, and older people, as is clearly evident with prescription drug misuse, the American population is shocked and outraged, searches desperately to understand the social issues that caused the problem, and advocates for sympathetic social responses rooted in drug treatment.

Although past-month prescription drug misuse is more common among blacks than whites, males than females, urban residents than rural residents, poor than wealthier Americans, and the less educated than the more educated in the United States, in the 2014 NSDUH the prescription drug misuse problem is newsworthy because the demographics groups that we do not expect to use drugs are disproportionately misusing prescription medications compared with other forms of drug use. The race, gender, urban versus rural, and education gaps in prescription drug misuse rates are much narrower for prescription drug misuse than for other drugs. Like urban school shootings that do not receive significant media attention because urban violence is expected in our culture, prescription drug misuse problems among demographic groups that our culture expects to have drug use problems are not newsworthy. On the other hand, just as rural school shootings receive massive media coverage because rural violence is unexpected, prescription drug misuse problems among demographic groups that are not viewed as traditional drug users generate considerable media coverage. The media coverage of the prescription drug misuse problem, most of which highlights stories of middle-class, white, female, and/or well-educated Americans, operates as an agenda-setting mechanism for the American public. Because prescription drug misuse among nonstereotypical drug using populations is newsworthy due to the rarity of drug use among these groups, the media covers the prescription drug misuse problem among these groups to attract consumers. Because the media covers the prescription drug misuse problem among these groups, the American public has come to view prescription drug misuse as a problem in need of immediate solutions.

Similar to the media coverage of sensationalized rural school shootings that attracted media readers, viewers, and listeners and led the American public to hold their elected officials accountable in their actions related to reducing (rural) school shootings, the American public has also been primed to hold elected officials accountable for solutions to the prescription drug misuse problem. The 2016 presidential election, especially the Republican primaries, provided ample evidence that addressing the prescription drug misuse problem was on the top of American voters' minds. As discussed earlier in the book, Chris Christie, candidate for the Republican nomination for president and governor of New Jersey, regularly told the story of his law school friend who became addicted to prescription opioids following back surgery and a legitimate opioid prescription in his calls for the government to work to reduce the prescription drug misuse problem. On the campaign trail Jeb Bush, another candidate for the Republican nomination for president and former governor of Florida, also described the addiction problems his daughter faced and claimed that solving the prescription drug misuse problem would be his top priority as president. During her campaign for the Republican nomination for president, Carly Fiorina also shared her story of losing her stepdaughter to a drug overdose and stressed the need for more drug treatment programs. Other candidates for the Republican nomination for president, including Donald Trump, John Kasich, and Ted Cruz, all spoke regularly about the prescription drug misuse problem on the campaign trail and published plans to address the problem. Hillary Clinton, the Democratic nominee for president in 2016, also published a detailed plan for how her administration would address the prescription drug misuse problem. As president of the United States, Barack Obama requested $1.1 billion to expand access to treatment for opioid addiction, which was not approved, and President Donald Trump established the President's Commission on Combating Drug Addiction and the Opioid Crisis and formally declared opioid abuse a public health emergency in 2017. There is even some evidence that counties with higher prescription opioid use rates were much more likely to vote for Trump than counties with lower prescription opioid use rates.[9] People with more familiarity with the devastating impact of prescription opioid misuse voted for Trump at much higher rates. There is thus recent evidence that the agenda setting and priming of the public by the media directly translated to votes for Trump in 2016.

Clearly, the public agenda established by the media coverage of the prescription drug misuse problem primed the American population to push politicians for solutions to the issue, but the framing of the prescription drug misuse problem by the media is also important. In stark contrast to the framing of the 1980s crack cocaine crisis that focused on the individual immorality of the poor urban minorities who were using crack, which correlated with the harsh criminal justice punishment response to the problem, the prescription drug misuse problem in the United States has largely been framed as a social structural problem. The entire "diseases of despair" narrative described earlier in this book, which focuses on the large-scale financial despair rooted in macroeconomic changes in the United States that have disproportionately impacted white men in mainly rural areas, is an example of how the prescription drug misuse problem has been framed in sociological, not individual, terms. The stories of celebrities and everyday Americans who struggle with prescription drug misuse presented earlier in the book are replete with questions as to why the person turned to prescription drug misuse, with possible answers ranging from excessive stress to peer influence and medical malfeasance. In fact, questions about the role of the medical profession in overprescribing addictive prescription medications is in and of itself a sociological explanation for the prescription drug misuse problem.

Given the apparent sociological framing of the prescription drug misuse problem in the United States, it is not surprising that the policy solutions that have been promoted by politicians have overwhelmingly stressed treatment over criminal justice punishments. A full description of the media portrayal of the prescription drug misuse problem is outside of the scope of this book. Answers to the original question posed in this book as to why politicians responded much more compassionately to the prescription drug misuse problem than to previous drug problems in the United States, namely crack, however, cannot ignore the demographic composition of prescription drug misuse or the media agenda setting, priming, or framing of the prescription drug misuse problem. Future research should include full-scale analyses of the media coverage of the prescription drug misuse problem to more accurately determine the degree to which media representations of the problem contributed to the treatment-based rather than punishment-based public responses.

What is clear, however, is that the prescription drug misuse problem in the United States has elicited compassionate political responses that largely ignore criminal justice sanctions and promote drug treatment and reforms to social institutions, including the medical profession. Most surprising, these compassionate solutions to the prescription drug problem have recently been promoted and supported by Republican politicians and the Republican Party, which is generally but not exclusively credited with promoting and implementing the harsh criminal justice approach to the crack scare of the 1980s. Forging a better understanding of the disparate policy solutions to the prescription drug misuse and crack problems in the United States should be a major focus of future research.

An Issue of Power?

Media representations of the prescription drug misuse problem in the United States have likely shaped the American public's reaction to the prescription drug misuse problem and their demands of elected leaders. What has not been adequately addressed throughout this book is the nature of power in our society and how power has likely contributed to public response to the prescription drug misuse problem. Social power is closely related to how the media chooses to portray a societal problem, but the conflict theory of criminology adds further contextualization to the public reactions and policy approaches.

Two different versions of the conflict theory in criminology are relevant to the prescription drug misuse problem in the United States. The legal reality theory, developed by William Chambliss, distinguishes between the *law on the books* and the *law in action*.[10] The law on the books, or written law, should apply to all citizens equally, but the law in action, or the way that authorities choose to enforce the law, tends to favor citizens with social and economic power. Stated simply, law enforcement officials (i.e., police, prosecutors, and judges) enforce the written laws in a way that serves the interests of the wealthy and powerful in a society and that controls the behaviors of the powerless. In other words, the written laws apply to all people in a society, but the enforcement of the laws targets specific populations who pose a threat to the people with power. The enforced laws develop from the principle of organizational imperative, which specifies that organizations structure actions to maximize reward and minimize trouble for the organizations. For law enforcement agencies, the reward to be gained is public support and the risk is withdrawal of public support, both of which are tied to funding for policing organizations. Law enforcement agencies therefore seek public and political support by focusing policing and arrest efforts on laws that are broken by powerless populations. Conversely, law enforcement also avoids enforcing the laws broken by the wealthy and powerful.

Laws that prohibit the misuse of prescription drugs apply to all Americans equally, but the manner in which those laws are applied in action is still in question. No publicly available data separates prescription drug misuse or illegal possession arrests from arrests for the use or possession of other drugs. To be sure, the media will present news reports of doctors who illegally prescribe controlled medications and drug traffickers caught with massive amounts of illegal prescription medications, and there is a current push by law enforcement to crack down on pain management clinics, but the arrest data for illegal use and/or possession of prescription medications will be much more telling as to how the law is operating in action. Based on current public sentiment in favor of increased access to drug treatment for prescription drug misusers, it is likely that the number of arrests for illegal prescription drug misuse or possession is low in comparison to the prevalence rate for prescription drug misuse. Additionally, based on demographic discrepancies in arrest rates for the possession of other drugs based on race, it is likely that the arrest rate for illegal prescription drug possession is low for whites in relation to whites' prescription drug misuse prevalence rate, which further highlights the difference between the law on the books and law in action. Marijuana use, for example, is nearly as prevalent among white Americans, but black Americans are arrested for simple marijuana possession more than three times more often than white Americans.[11] Clearly, the law in action is much different from the law on the books for marijuana possession, with minorities arrested at disproportionately higher rates than whites. Accordingly, the law in action for illegal possession of prescription medications is likely applied disproportionately to minorities than whites. Future research should fully investigate the discrepancies in arrest rates for illegal prescription drug possession between powerful and powerless groups in the United States. That said, based on arrest discrepancies that have been documented for other drugs, it would be shocking if whites, wealthier people, and college-educated Americans were arrested at rates that are anywhere near comparable to prevalence use rates among those groups.

The other conflict perspective that is applicable to the prescription drug misuse problem in the United States is Richard Quinney's theory of the social reality of crime.[12] The main impetus of the theory is that people with power make laws that control the behaviors of those who could threaten their power and that the powerful direct the actions of law enforcement agencies to mitigate the threats to their social and economic power. Throughout the process of lawmaking and directing the ways in which the law is applied in action, the result is that society adopts an ideology of crime that maintains the power of the social and economic elites in society. Most important to the prescription drug misuse problem in the United States is the belief that powerless populations are dangerous drug users and should therefore be arrested, prosecuted, and imprisoned for drug use, thereby creating the image that drug use is not prevalent or dangerous among powerful groups and therefore not in need of criminal justice attention. The best illustration of Quinney's social reality of crime is the historical difference in mandatory minimum sentences associated with crack and powder cocaine. Often referred to as the 100:1 rule, people needed to possess 100 times more powder cocaine than crack cocaine to receive the same mandatory minimum sentence. In the late 1970s and early 1980s when the sentencing guidelines were developed, white Americans were mainly using cocaine in powder form, but black Americans were using cocaine in crack form. In their enforcement of cocaine laws the police therefore targeted black populations, resulting in a rapid growth in black Americans being imprisoned for cocaine crimes. The increased incarceration rate of black Americans for cocaine offenses in turn justified the targeting of black Americans for cocaine and other drug crimes and contributed to the perception that cocaine was a major problem among black Americans.[13] This whole process occurred during a time in which there was no evidence whatsoever that cocaine use was more prevalent or causing more problems among black Americans than white Americans, with the notable exception of the violence that surrounded the crack cocaine trade. The result, however, was that Americans developed an ideology of crime that supported the wildly disparate sentencing for cocaine, based on whether it was in powder form (less punishment) or crack form (more punishment), an ideology that clearly protected the interests of white Americans to the detriment to black Americans.

As described earlier in the book, history is replete with examples of powerful groups using drug laws to protect their interests against threats from less powerful groups. Marijuana, for example, was criminalized as a way to deport Mexican immigrants who provided labor during the westward expansion of the United States when their labor was no longer beneficial to powerful white Americans.[14] Like the comparison of arrest rates for the illegal possession of prescription medications being in need of research, future research should also compare the criminal punishments associated with the illegal possession of prescription medications compared with punishments for the possession of other drugs. Based on the social reality of crime, because prescription drug misuse is a disproportionately bigger problem than other drugs among white Americans, criminal sanctions for the illegal possession of prescription drugs are likely less severe than criminal sanctions for the possession of other drugs. More important, however, public and political reactions to the prescription drug misuse problem in the United States are more sympathetic, more concerned with the social causes of the problem, and more in favor of treatment solutions than criminal justice interventions than has occurred with any other drug problem in U.S. history. Public perceptions of prescription drug misuse are especially surprising given the dramatic, devastating, and deadly consequences of prescription drug abuse in the United States.

Could the more sympathetic perception of prescription drug misusers be related to the fact that prescription drug misuse is more white, more middle class, and more college-educated than other forms of drug use? We strongly suspect that this is the case, but future research will need to empirically examine this proposition. An important analogue to the prescription drug misuse problem in the United States that can help us understand the differential reaction to prescription drug misuse based on social power is America's experience with marijuana. When marijuana was primarily a drug among minority populations in the United States, it was criminalized, strongly enforced, and punished harshly. But as marijuana has become increasingly prevalent in white middle-class and college-educated populations, states have moved to decriminalize and even legalize the recreational use of marijuana. Given the distressing number of deaths associated with prescription drug misuse and the media and political attention given to prescription drug misuse deaths, it is unlikely that states will move to decriminalize prescription drug misuse. The relative normalization, sympathy, and lack of criminal justice emphasis associated with the prescription drug misuse problem in the United States, however, strongly illustrates the degree to which Americans have internalized an ideology that "real" drug use is a dangerous problem among the powerless in need of punishment, while prescription drug misuse among dominant groups is a problem that deserves sympathy and criminal justice lenience.

The Prescription Drug Death, Not Misuse, Epidemic

Throughout this book, we have investigated nearly every minute detail in the prescription drug misuse prevalence rate statistics in an attempt to find evidence that the United States is experiencing, or has experienced in the past, a prescription drug *misuse* epidemic. Despite our best efforts, we simply do not find that the United States as a whole or any subgroup in the United States is experiencing, or has experienced in the past, a prescription drug *misuse* epidemic. Although U.S. culture has a long history of decrying any level of drug use as an epidemic and although the term "epidemic" is colloquially used to describe any problem that is in need of immediate public intervention, the prescription drug misuse patterns in the United States over the past 20 years show no evidence of reaching epidemic levels by any standard definition of an epidemic, including the Centers for Disease Control and Prevention's (CDC) official definition. Prescription drug misuse rates in the United States are relatively low and have been decreasing for a long period of time. Although some groups have experienced more pronounced increases in prescription drug misuse at different periods over the past 20 years, most notably young noncollege white men living in rural areas, those groups have also shown recent and substantial declines in prescription drug misuse rates. Stated concisely, the United States is not experiencing a prescription drug *misuse* epidemic. Based on all available evidence scrutinized throughout this book, the public reaction to the prescription drug misuse problem in the United States is best summarized by a comment from the late comedian Richard Pryor, who once famously stated that "They call it an epidemic now. That means white folks are doing it." Pryor was referencing crack cocaine, but the same sentiment, altered to include other powerful groups, can be applied to the current prescription drug misuse problem in the United States.

Although prescription drug *misuse* is not an epidemic in the United States, prescription drug misuse *deaths* are an epidemic. Even as prescription drug misuse prevalence rates have declined in recent years, prescription drug misuse deaths have continued to rapidly increase. The prescription drug overdose death rate in the United States tripled between 1999 and 2014. Between 2002 and 2014, where comparable rates of prescription drug misuse are available, the prescription drug overdose death rate more than doubled, but the prevalence of past-year prescription drug misuse declined by 11 percent. Prescription drug misuse therefore has become much deadlier among a shrinking population of misusers. Prescription opioid misuse dominates the prescription drug overdose statistics, with opioids responsible for 73 percent of all prescription drug overdose deaths in 2014. Further, the prescription opioid overdose death rate more than tripled between 1999 and 2014, and prescription opioid overdose deaths increased by 127 percent from 2002 to 2014, when the prevalence of past-year prescription opioid misuse decreased by 35 percent. The prescription drug misuse death epidemic is primarily a prescription opioid overdose death epidemic, although deaths from benzodiazepines have been increasing rapidly in recent years too. As the percentage of the population who misuses prescription medications, especially opioids, dwindles, death rates have continued to skyrocket. Prescription drug misuse deaths, not misuse rates, are an epidemic in need of immediate and significant public attention by any definition of the term.

When the deadly consequences of prescription drug misuse are considered independent of the misuse prevalence rates, the strong public and political reaction to the prescription drug misuse problem in the United States and the emphasis on public health rather than criminal justice solutions appear to be in line with the scope and nature of the problem. The mortality data, however, highlight the expected versus unexpected dynamics that drive public and political reactions described above to a stronger degree than the misuse prevalence data. For instance, whereas prescription drug misuse is equally prevalent among black and white Americans, prescription drug misuse overdose death rates are more than twice as common among white Americans (10.7 deaths per 100,000 white Americans, 4.5 per 100,000 black Americans in 2014). Additionally, the prescription drug misuse overdose death rates were slightly higher in rural areas than in urban areas in 2014, a result of the much faster increases in the prescription drug misuse overdose death rates in rural areas than in urban areas between 1999 and 2014. Similarly, the prescription drug overdose death rate among males remained higher than the rate among females in 2014, but the prescription drug misuse overdose death rate among females increased much more quickly among females between 1999 and 2014. Just as the demographics of prescription drug misuse defy traditional assumptions of drug use patterns in the United States and therefore generate newsworthiness, the demographic patterns and trends of prescription drug misuse overdose deaths suggest that deaths related to prescription drugs have strongly afflicted "unexpected" groups.

The prescription drug mortality problems among "unexpected" populations equates to increased media coverage, agenda setting, and priming. Prescription drug overdose deaths are an obvious and growing epidemic in need of public health solutions in the United States, but the implications of the unexpected demographic mortality patterns for the scale and nature of the public and political response to the prescription drug misuse overdose death problem cannot be ignored. Prescription drug misuse deaths have devastated all groups across the United States, but whites, females, and rural residents have been hit particularly hard by this growing epidemic. Unfortunately, mortality data by income levels is not available from the CDC. Future research should fully investigate trends in prescription drug misuse deaths by income.

As prescription drug misuse mortality rates have increased in recent years while prescription drug misuse prevalence rates have decreased, it is clear that prescription drug misuse has become increasingly deadly among a smaller and smaller group of users. This means that this small and shrinking group of prescription drug misusers are using greater quantities of prescription drugs, misusing prescription drugs at a higher frequency, ingesting prescription drugs in a more dangerous manner (i.e., injecting), and/or misusing prescription medications laced with more deadly substances. The limited available evidence does suggest that this small group of chronic prescription drug misusers, especially prescription opioid misusers, misuses large amounts of prescription medications at a high frequency and that the small group of chronic prescription opioid misusers is likely to also use heroin. A concerted research effort that addresses the high frequency, high dosage, chronic prescription drug, and opioid misuser population is needed, however, to better connect shrinking misuse rates to the growing mortality rates.

Despite questions about the frequency, dosage, and dangerous methods of ingesting illegal prescription medications, it is obvious that fentanyl and other synthetic opioids have been a major force behind growing opioid-related mortality rates in the United States, prescription or otherwise. Of the 52,404 total overdose deaths in the United States in 2015, fentanyl and other synthetic opioids were implicated in 9,580 overdose deaths. About 18 percent of all overdose deaths, or 39 percent of all opioid-related deaths, in 2015 were related to fentanyl or other synthetic opioids. Further, fentanyl and other synthetic opioid-related deaths have increased faster than any other category of overdose deaths from 1999 to 2015. Whereas the total overdose death rate in the United States has nearly tripled over this period, the fentanyl and other synthetic opioid overdose death rate increased by 1,140 percent from 1999 to 2015. Synthetic opioids, including fentanyl, are clearly implicated in the rising overdose death rates in the United States. When synthetic opioids are removed from the overdose death statistics, however, prescription opioid-related overdose deaths still increased by 150 percent from 1999 to 2015. Fentanyl is part of the increasing deadliness of prescription drug misuse, but prescription drug misuse, especially prescription opioid misuse, has increased dramatically independent of fentanyl and other synthetic opioids.

Although the study presented in this book was limited to the data available at the time the analyses were conducted and data from years that allowed for comparisons between misuse rates and overdose death rates, the CDC has since released overdose death information from 2016 and estimates from 2017. Overdose death rates continued to rise dramatically in 2016, increasing an additional 21 percent between 2015 and 2016 to 63,600 overdose deaths. Synthetic opioid-related overdose deaths, including fentanyl, doubled from 2015 to 2016. Heroin-related deaths also increased from 2015 to 2016 (a 20 percent increase), albeit more slowly than the increases in overdose deaths attributed to synthetic opioids. Prescription opioid overdose deaths increased by 13 percent between 2015 and 2016. Notably, between 2015 and 2016, synthetic opioids became the leading cause of opioid-related overdose deaths in the United States for the first time, accounting for 6.2 deaths per 100,000 people in 2016, compared with overdose death rates of 4.9 and 4.4 per 100,000 people for heroin and prescription opioids in 2016, respectively.[15] Preliminary results from the 2017 overdose death data released by the CDC estimate 72,287 overdose deaths in that year, an additional 14 percent increase from the 2016 statistics. The data estimate nearly 30,000 overdose deaths attributed to synthetic opioids in 2017, an additional increase of 9,000 synthetic opioid overdose deaths from the prior year, but deaths from heroin and prescription opioids remained relatively unchanged from 2016 to 2017. Fentanyl and other synthetic opioids have entered the prescription opioid and heroin markets and have come to dominate the overdose death epidemic in the United States.[16]

Future research will need to address the demographic factors associated with fentanyl misuse and investigate patterns of intentional versus unintentional fentanyl misuse. Unfortunately, the NSDUH does not include questions about fentanyl misuse. Anecdotal evidence suggests that many of the fentanyl-related overdose deaths resulted from unintentional fentanyl ingestion, meaning that the heroin or misused prescription opioids were unknowingly cut with fentanyl to increase the high achieved by the drug at a low cost. On the other hand, reports are starting to emerge that a small number of Americans are intentionally abusing fentanyl and other synthetic opioids to achieve strong euphoric effects, but the potency of synthetic opioids is so strong that minor variations in the concentration of fentanyl can have deadly consequences. Fentanyl and other synthetic opioids therefore must be the focus of future research on the prescription drug misuse problem and overdose death epidemic in the United States.

Conclusions on the U.S. Prescription Drug Misuse Problem

As highlighted by the new information on prescription drug overdose deaths described above that has been published since we began the research presented throughout the book, the prescription drug misuse and death problem in the United States is an evolving issue. The United

States is currently in the midst of the prescription drug death crisis, and new information is constantly becoming available that can change our interpretations of the problem. This book, however, set out to understand the prescription drug misuse problem in the United States from a historical perspective and to capture the current state of the problem within data that was available at the time the research began. The overall goal was to understand why the prescription drug misuse problem in the United States has received a much different public and political response than prior drug crises in the United States.

Based on the prescription drug misuse data over the past 20 years, the comparable overdose death data over the past 15 years, and the available literature from prior drug use crises in the United States, we can make several tentative conclusions about the current U.S. prescription drug misuse problem.

- First, because rates of prescription drug misuse are comparatively low and have been decreasing in recent years, the misuse of prescription medications is not a national epidemic. Prescription drug misuse prevalence rates are certainly more problematic among specific groups in the United States, and misuse rates are much higher than prevalence rates for hard drug use, but the groups in which prescription drug misuse has historically been concentrated are experiencing prevalence rate decreases alongside the rest of the U.S. population.
- Second, although prescription drug *misuse* is not a national epidemic, prescription drug-related overdose *deaths* are a national crisis of epidemic proportions. Overdose deaths, primarily related to prescription opioid overdoses, have continued to skyrocket in recent years even as misuse prevalence rates have declined, meaning that the overdose deaths are coming from shrinking numbers of prescription drug misusers. The United States has experienced a prolonged prescription drug misuse era that has culminated in a prescription drug misuse overdose death epidemic.
- Third, the demographic patterns of prescription drug misuse and overdose death are different from similar patterns with other drugs. The "unexpected" groups of people who are disproportionately afflicted by prescription drug misuse and death have likely driven the intense media and political attention given to the prescription drug misuse and death problem in the United States. This is not to say that the massive media and political response to the prescription drug misuse and death problem and the focus on treatment rather than incarceration are unwarranted; rather, it is clear that prior drug crises in the United States received much different media and political responses, because those drug problems afflicted expected drug-using populations, populations with less social and economic power than the demographic populations that have been disproportionately involved in

prescription drug misuse and death. A public health approach that includes a focus on harm reduction, similar to what has been implemented in reaction to the current prescription drug misuse and death crisis in the United States, would have been better suited to address the prior drug use problems in the United States (i.e., crack) than the criminal justice punishment-driven approach that was employed to address those prior drug use problems.

- Fourth, the public health solutions that have been implemented in response to the prescription drug misuse and death problem have primarily targeted the misuse of prescription opioids. The treatment and prevention solutions have shown varying degrees of success, but because there has not been a federal policy program to address the problem so far, comparative analyses of what works are not possible. States and local governments have implemented different prevention and drug treatment strategies, and the differences between the programs make it difficult to identify the most effective policies and practices to address the prescription drug misuse and death problem. A fully funded federal policy strategy needs to implemented immediately across the country so that researchers and policy makers can more accurately understand what works to reduce problems of prescription drug misuse and death.
- Fifth, opioids—whether prescription, synthetic, or heroin—are the primary substance involved in the current drug use crisis in the United States, and the existing policies focus almost exclusively focus on preventing the use of and overdose deaths from opioids. The focus on opioids is reasonable, considering that opioid abuse in all forms dominates both the misuse and death statistics. Policies, however, need to account for the varying reasons that people misuse and abuse opioids. There are some people who misuse and abuse opioids following legitimate medical opioid use that led to addiction, whereas others misuse and abuse opioids following youthful experimentation, and a small group of Americans have incorporated opioids into their existing dangerous drug use habits. Each group will likely respond differently to different forms of treatment and prevention, but research has yet to distinguish treatment and prevention efforts to reduce opioid misuse and abuse based on the different underlying motivations for use.
- Sixth, the current treatment and prevention programs that have been implemented in a variety of forms across the United States, almost all of which have been at the state and local levels, in recent years have mainly focused on the immediate concerns of treating addictions, preventing diversion and trafficking, and preventing overdose deaths (i.e., Narcan). No large-scale strategy to address the prescription drug misuse and death problem has addressed the sociological factors that underlie prescription drug misuse and death. High levels of social strain, low levels of social control, and strong peer and family influence drive much of the prescription drug misuse problem in the United States. To be effective, future treatment and prevention

efforts must address the underlying sociological causes of misuse and abuse. Other macrolevel factors that might be associated with prescription drug misuse and death, such as income inequality that has caused widespread despair among certain populations in the United States, need to be investigated in future research and addressed in policy solutions.

Hope and Resilience

Despite the barrage of distressing information on the trends and consequences of prescription drug misuse in the United States described throughout this book and presented ubiquitously in the media and political coverage of the prescription drug misuse and death problem in the United States, there are many reasons to be hopeful about the future of prescription drug misuse and death. Stories of hope, resilience, and recovery are becoming more common in media representations of the prescription drug misuse problem. A 2014 CNN news story, for instance, told of a woman named Cynthia, a suburban middle-class grandmother of 18 who struggled with prescription opioid and heroin addiction for over a decade. Like so many media depictions of prescription drug misuse among middle-class Americans, Cynthia had a great life until a doctor prescription OxyContin to treat pain associated with multiple cesarean section births. Nearly 10 years of addiction to opioid medications and heroin followed, destroying her marriage and family until she hit rock bottom and her mother checked her into a 30-day inpatient rehabilitation program. At the time the CNN article was written, Cynthia had been clean for three years, had remarried, and had a good job managing more than 200 employees at a credit card company, and her grandchildren once again began visiting her.[17]

The *New York Times* also reported the success story of a famous photographer, Nam Goldin, in a 2018 exposé. Goldin's path to prescription opioid addiction resembles the all too common tale of experiencing wrist pain that was treated medically with OxyContin and escalated into heroin and fentanyl abuse. After years of opioid addiction, Goldin experience a near-fatal overdose from a mixture of heroin and fentanyl. The overdose motivated him to seek treatment at an inpatient treatment center, where she resided for more than two months. Goldin is now clean and using her addiction experiences to organize a group whose mission is to demand that museums reject funding from Purdue Pharma, the manufacturer of OxyContin, and push Purdue to instead fund rehabilitation and treatment centers, advertise the dangers of prescription opioids, and educate doctors on the risks of overprescribing opioid medications.[18]

Similarly, a story of a middle-class, middle-age woman named Rachelle was published in the *Kansas City Star* newspaper in 2016. Like the vast majority of prescription drug misuse stories, Rachelle was prescribed Vicodin after a tubal ligation reversal surgery that left her in severe pain. She became physically addicted to Vicodin and resorted to doctor shopping for more pills and began conning family members out of their pain medications. After years of prescription opioid medication addiction that destroyed her life and family, she tried methadone treatment, but methadone was not enough, and her life derailed again, further complicated by an additional surgery and more opioid prescriptions. After additional years of addiction, failed treatment attempts, homelessness, and a series of arrests, Rachelle finally decided that she needed to quit misusing prescription opioids for good. She began an outpatient treatment program that focuses on mental health counseling to assist in her sobriety. At the time of the news story, Rachelle had been clean for about two years, had rebuilt relationships with her children, had her own apartment, and had a job at a local restaurant.[19]

In addition to the individual success stories that inspire hope for the future of prescription drug misuse in the United States, many communities have also had success is curbing prescription drug misuse and death. A 2018 *New York Times* report, for instance, highlights Dayton, Ohio, as an example of a community that is beginning to recover from the prescription drug misuse problem and death epidemic. By using a multipronged emergency response strategy funded by both federal and state grants that focused on expanding access to Narcan, providing drug treatment to city and county prisoners, building additional capacity for drug treatment programs across the county, and implementing further mechanisms to control opioid overprescribing, the county reports that overdose deaths and emergency room visits decreased by more than 60 percent in a one-year period.[20]

Other cities across the United States are starting to document that harm-reduction strategies are working to mitigate the negative consequences of prescription drug misuse. Scott County, Indiana, for instance, began a needle-exchange program in reaction to a steep increase in the county's HIV infection rate in 2015. Although aimed primarily at heroin users, the program also helped to reduce the harms associated with intravenous prescription drug misuse. Besides reducing the transmission of HIV and other blood-borne diseases spread through sharing needles, the program also used the needle-exchange program as an initial point of contact with drug addicts for the county health department with the hope that the contact would be the initial step in providing drug treatment and HIV testing for the addicts. After three years of the county running the needle-exchange program, the CDC reported that the percentage of drug users who shared needles in Scott County decreased from 74 percent to 22 percent. Additionally, HIV testing increased dramatically in the county, and nearly all addicts who tested positive for HIV stopped sharing needles. The most important outcome of the needle-exchange program in Scott County, Indiana, could possibly be that the program reduced the stigma of addiction, leading to an increase in the numbers of addicts seeking treatment.[21] Charleston, West Virginia, has recently restarted a similar need exchange program.

Another unique and potentially effective strategy in fighting the prescription drug misuse and death problem in the United States was recently implemented in Tempe, Arizona. By testing the city's wastewater for traces of prescription medications and street drugs such as heroin, the city is able to monitor the impact of crackdowns on pill mills and target specific areas of the city that show spikes in concentrations of prescription medications that are often misused. Wastewater can be quickly tested for overall concentrations of specific drug compounds, and city authorities can use the near real-time data to prepare emergency officials to target certain communities in the city with large doses of Narcan to address potential overdoses. For example, if a pain clinic is shut down or raided by law enforcement, wastewater can determine if those addicts whose access to prescription opioids was cut off are turning to heroin or fentanyl to feed their addictions. Importantly, the wastewater testing can pinpoint the specific areas of the city that are showing dangerous increases in opioid use and direct resources to prevent deaths and provide clean needles to prevent the spread of diseases. The effectiveness of the wastewater programs has not been empirically assessed, but the potential of wastewater-monitoring programs in reducing the harms of prescription drug misuse (and other forms of opioid use) is so great that many other cities, including Louisville, Kentucky, are considering the implementation of similar programs.[22]

Data-driven solutions are beginning to show success in addressing the prescription drug misuse and overdose death problems in cities across the country. Although needle-exchange programs and wastewater-monitoring systems are harm-reduction strategies, not necessarily designed to effectively reduce the rate of prescription drug misuse in the cities, curbing the prescription drug death epidemic is an important first step. Multipronged approaches that include treatment, counseling, an increased availability of Narcan, and diversion reductions are also showing successes in reducing deaths and emergency room visits for prescription drug and other opioid overdoses, but there is no evidence that prescription drug misuse rates are decreasing in those areas. Access to effective treatment, however, will likely decrease prescription drug misuse prevalence rates too.

Another potential strategy for reducing the harms associated with prescription drug abuse has been shown as a collateral consequence of Colorado's legalization of marijuana. In their study published in the *American Journal of Public Health,* Livingston and colleagues reported that the legalization of recreational cannabis was associated with a decrease in opioid-related overdose deaths by 0.7 per month. The reduction in opioid overdose deaths in Colorado after implementing the legal use and sale of cannabis products for recreational use was statistically significant and was maintained after controlling for many relevant variables. The finding therefore suggests that the legalization of marijuana did influence reductions in overdose deaths, at least over the short-term. The authors caution that more research is needed to validate the effect of marijuana legalization in reducing the harms associated with prescription drug misuse, but the results are certainly promising.[23] As more states legalize recreational marijuana, additional data will show if legal marijuana reduces overdose deaths in other states. At this point, however, it is certainly possible that legal access to marijuana provides opioid misusers a legal alternative to pain reduction and a way to manage the physical withdrawal symptoms associated with stopping opioid use. States that are working to reduce drug overdose deaths and prescription opioid abuse would be well served to examine the positive and unintentional outcomes of Colorado's experiment with marijuana legalization.

As we described earlier in the book and reinforced throughout the presentation of the data, the United States appears to have experienced an extended prescription drug use era that escalated in the mid-1990s and began to subside in the early 2000s. We contend that rather than viewing the prescription drug misuse problem in the United States as an epidemic, as that word carries harsh meanings that legitimize punitive criminal justice approaches that often exacerbate drug problems, we are better served by describing the prescription drug misuse problem as a drug era. The data clearly show that a small number of people in the early and mid-1990s began misusing prescription medications, which characterizes the incubation phase described by Golub and colleagues. The expansion phase occurred in the late 1990s and early 2000s, as prescription drugs became more available (spurred by the introduction of OxyContin) and spread into traditional drug-using populations. The plateau phase encompassed most of the 2000s, when everybody who had an interest in prescription drug misuse and had access to illegal prescription medications misused prescription drugs, especially adolescents. The United States, however, has been in a prolonged decline phase for the past several years whereby the popularity of prescription drug use has subsided, possibly based on public education projects designed to stigmatize and highlight the harms of prescription drug misuse.

As Golub and associates explained, however, as prevalence use rates in a population decrease during the decline phase of a drug era, many of the most addicted will continue to use the drug. We contend that the strong addictive qualities of some prescription medications, especially prescription opioids, have created a context in which the prescription drug misusers who continue use are the high-dosage, high-frequency addicted misusers. Casual prescription drug misusers have abandoned prescription drug misuse as the drug era has subsided, but those misusers who remain are strongly connected to prescription drug misuse through addiction. Prescription drug misusers who have continued this drug use pattern throughout the decline phase are likely responsible for the rapidly increasing prescription drug overdose rates, likely through a combination of higher-frequency, higher-dosage misuse; the introduction of more dangerous substances (i.e., fentanyl) into the illegal prescription drug market; and transitions away from prescription opioids to heroin. As the nation continues to combat the deadly effects of prescription drug misuse—and the disturbing trend of transitioning from prescription opioid misuse to heroin use—the good news is that the data show that the United States is clearly in the decline phase of the prescription drug misuse era.

Further highlighting the good news about the prescription drug misuse problem in the United States is that youths, whose drug use patterns are predictive of future nationwide drug use trends, have shown significant declines in prescription drug misuse prevalence rates in recent years. Youths are rapidly moving away from prescription drug misuse, so if the past drug use trends continue to be predictive of future nationwide drug use trends, the United States will likely see continued declines in prescription drug misuse over the next decade. Nationwide trends in prescription drug misuse are already beginning to show that most Americans are moving away from prescription drug misuse, and declines in prescription drug misuse among young people in the United States portends good news for the future of prescription drug misuse in the United States. The one issue that needs to be closely monitored is the recent evidence that as Americans have moved away from prescription opioid misuse, many have turned to heroin.

The last piece of evidence that provides at least a glimpse of hope is that the latest projections from the CDC show that overdose deaths from prescription opioid medications appear to have stopped increasing from 2016 to 2017 in the United States and might in fact be showing signs of decreasing. The President's Commission on Combating Drug Addiction and the Opioid Crisis is an indicator that the federal government is moving toward a national policy strategy to reduce prescription drug misuse, and funding is slowly becoming available. The United States is moving in the right direction, and all available evidence presents an optimistic outlook that the worst of the prescription drug misuse problem has passed.

Notes

Introduction

1. Craig Reinarman and Harry G. Levine, eds., *Crack in America: Demon Drugs and Social Justice* (Berkeley: University of California Press, 1997), 1.
2. Harry G. Levine, "The Alcohol Problem in America: From Temperance to Alcoholism," *British Journal of Addiction* 79 (1984): 109–119.
3. Reinarman and Levine, *Crack in America*, 6.
4. David F. Musto, *The American Disease: Origins of Narcotic Control* (New Haven, CT: Yale University Press).
5. Reinarman and Levine, *Crack in America*, 19.
6. Ibid., 18.
7. Ibid.
8. Ibid., 21.
9. Michael Massing, "What Ever Happened to the 'War on Drugs?'," *New York Review of Books*, June 11, 1992, https://www.nybooks.com/articles/1992/06/11/what-ever-happened-to-the-war-on-drugs/.
10. *National Household Survey on Drug Abuse: Population Estimates, 1992* (Washington, DC: National Institute on Drug Abuse).
11. Reinarman and Levine, *Crack in America*, 32–33.
12. Keith Harriston and Sally Jenkins, "Maryland Basketball Star Len Bias Is Dead at 22," *Washington Post*, June 20, 1986.
13. Michael Goodwin, "Drug Charges Seen in Death of Bias," *New York Times*, July 20, 1986.
14. Sam McMantis, "When Rights Go Wrong: Before June 27 Drug Death, Don Rogers Was Troubled; Maybe He Cared Too Much," *Los Angeles Times*, August 3, 1986.
15. Emanuella Grinberg, "Prince's Death: The Latest," CNN, June 3, 2016, https://www.cnn.com/2016/05/04/entertainment/prince-death-latest/index.html.

16. "Fentanyl," Drug Enforcement Administration, https://www.dea.gov/sites/default/files/sites/getsmartaboutdrugs.com/files/publications/DoA_2017Ed_Updated_6.16.17.pdf#page=40.

17. Faith Karimi and Sara Sidner, "Feds Seeking Answers on How Prince Got Fentanyl, the Opioid That Killed Him," CNN, May 4, 2016, https://www.cnn.com/2016/06/03/health/prince-death-opioid-overdose/index.html.

18. "Ledger's Death Caused by Accidental Overdose," CNN, February 6, 2008. http://www.cnn.com/2008/SHOWBIZ/Movies/02/06/heath.ledger/.

19. Shawn Adler, "Heath Ledger Battled Drug Addiction, Source Confirms to MTV News," MTV, January 31, 2008, http://www.mtv.com/news/1580725/heath-ledger-battled-drug-addiction-source-confirms-to-mtv-news.

20. Erin Coulehan, "Michael Jackson Was a Drug Addict, AEG Expert Testifies," *Rolling Stone,* August 28, 2013, https://www.rollingstone.com/music/music-news/michael-jackson-was-a-drug-addict-aeg-expert-testifies-118882/.

21. Jen Chaney, "The Full Story on Michael Jackson's Tragic Death," *Washington Post,* June 14, 2013, https://www.washingtonpost.com/entertainment/books/the-full-story-on-michael-jacksons-tragic-death/2016/06/14/5d9f74ee-3181-11e6-8758-d58e76e11b12_story.html?utm_term=.919f39fc3483.

22. Matt Hamilton, "Michael Jackson's Ex-Wife Offers Window into Singer's Drug Abuse," *Los Angeles Times,* August 14, 2013, http://www.latimes.com/local/lanow/la-me-ln-debbie-rowe-testifies-michael-jackson-death-20130814-story.html.

23. Chris Baltimore, "Coroner Says Jackson Died from Lethal Dose of Propofol," Reuters, August 28, 2009, https://www.reuters.com/article/us-jackson/jackson-had-lethal-levels-of-propofol-report-idUSTRE57G4W020090824.

24. Linda Lee Cadwell, "The Truth behind Life and Death of Bruce Lee," *Los Angeles Times,* August 17, 1998, http://articles.latimes.com/1998/aug/17/entertainment/ca-13848.

25. Edecio Martinez, "Brittany Murphy Death (Photos): Toxic Drug Combination Likely Killed Her, Expert Tells CBS," CBS News, December 22, 2009, https://www.cbsnews.com/news/brittany-murphy-death-photos-toxic-drug-combination-likely-killed-her-expert-tells-cbs/.

26. Richard Winton, "Corey Haim Obtained 553 Pills before He Died," *Los Angeles Times,* April 6, 2010, http://articles.latimes.com/2010/apr/06/local/la-me-corey-haim7-2010apr07.

27. Richard Winton, "Autopsy Finds Child Actor Corey Haim Died of Pneumonia," *Los Angeles Times,* May 5, 2010, http://articles.latimes.com/2010/may/05/local/la-me-0505-corey-haim-20100505.

28. "Whitney Houston Coroner's Report Details Drug Signs, Liquor, Drowning," CBS News, February 13, 2012, https://www.cbsnews.com/news/whitney-houston-coroners-report-details-drug-signs-liquor-drowning/.

29. Kim Carollo, "Whitney Houston's Death: Substance Abuse May Have Played a Role," ABC News, February 13, 2012, https://abcnews.go.com/Health/substance-abuse-played-role-whitney-houstons-death-experts/story?id=15568992.

30. Tony Fletcher, *Dear Boy: The Life of Keith Moon* (New York: Omnibus, 1998).

31. "Judy Garland, 47, Star of Stage and Screen, Is Found Dead in Her London Home," *New York Times*, June 23, 1969, https://archive.nytimes.com/www.nytimes.com/learning/general/onthisday/bday/0610.html?scp=1&sq=judy%2520garland%2520obituary&st=cse.

32. Gerald Clarke, *Get Happy: The Life of Judy Garland* (New York: Random House, 2001).

33. Anne-Marie O'Neill, "Seeking Serenity," *People*, June 7, 1999, https://people.com/archive/seeking-serenity-vol-51-no-21/.

34. Howard Markel, "Column: Marilyn Monroe and the Prescription Drugs That Killed Her," PBS, August 5, 2016, https://www.pbs.org/newshour/health/marilyn-monroe-and-the-prescription-drugs-that-killed-her.

35. Lois Banner, *Marilyn: The Passion and the Paradox* (New York: Bloomsbury, 2012).

36. Lindsay Kimble, "Elvis' Stepbrother Reveals the King's Drug Addiction Almost Caused Him to Choke to Death," *People*, July 22, 2016, https://people.com/celebrity/elvis-presleys-stepbrother-reveals-the-kings-final-years/.

37. Peter Guralnick, *Careless Love: The Unmaking of Elvis Presley* (Boston: Back Bay Books, 1999).

38. Ibid.

39. Reinarman and Levine, *Crack in America*.

40. Laura Ungar, "Mother Battles Pill Scourge That Claimed Son," *Courier Journal*, August 27, 2016, https://www.courier-journal.com/story/news/local/2016/08/27/mother-battles-pill-scourge-claimed-son/88568172/.

41. Ibid.

42. Ibid.

43. www.medicineabuseproject.com.

44. Ibid.

45. Ibid.

46. Ibid.

47. Ibid.

48. *Oxyana*, directed by Sean Dunne, 2013.

49. Jim Axelrod and Ashley Velie, "Drug Distributors under Fire in West Virginia Painkiller Epidemic," CBS News, January 7, 2016, https://www.cbsnews.com/news/drug-distributors-under-fire-in-west-virginia-painkiller-epidemic/.

50. Eric Eyre, "Flooded with Pain Pills, a WV Town Strikes Back against Drug Distributors," *West Virginia Gazette*, January 31, 2017, https://www.wvgazettemail.com/news/cops_and_courts/flooded-with-pain-pills-a-wv-town-strikes-back-against/article_e0831996-f5be-5fd9-8908-049838bdf38e.html.

51. Vince Beiser, "Prescription for Death: How Painkillers Destroyed the Town of War, WV," *Playboy*, March 17, 2014, https://playboysfw.kinja.com/precription-for-death-how-painkillers-destroyed-the-to-1544288108.

52. Joel Achenbach, "'No Longer 'Mayberry': A Small Ohio City Fights and Epidemic of Self-Destruction," *Washington Post*, December 29, 2016, https://www

.washingtonpost.com/national/health-science/no-longer-mayberry-a-small-ohio-city-fights-an-epidemic-of-self-destruction/2016/12/29/a95076f2-9a01-11e6-b3c9-f662adaa0048_story.html?utm_term=.c5afb9abcac2.

53. Ibid.

54. Harriet Ryan, Scott Glover, and Lisa Girion, "How Black-Market OxyContin Spurred a Town's Descent into Crime, Addiction and Heartbreak," *Los Angeles Times*, July 10, 2016, http://www.latimes.com/projects/la-me-oxycontin-everett/.

55. Harriet Ryan, Scott Glover, and Lisa Girion, "How Black-Market Oxycontin Spurred a Town's Descent into Crime, Addiction and Heartbreak," *Los Angeles Times*, July 10, 2016, http://www.latimes.com/projects/la-me-oxycontin-everett/.

56. *Under the Counter: The Diversion and Abuse of Controlled Prescription Drugs in the U.S.* (Washington, DC: National Center on Addiction and Substance Abuse, 2005).

57. Ibid.

58. Ibid.

59. Ibid.

60. Arthur Hughes, Matthew R. Williams, Rachel N. Lipari, Jonaki Bose, Elizabeth A. P. Copello, and Larry A. Kroutil, *Prescription Drug Use and Misuse in the United States: Results from the 2015 National Survey on Drug Use and Health* (Washington, DC: Substance Abuse and Mental Health Services Administration, 2015), https://www.samhsa.gov/data/sites/default/files/NSDUH-FFR2-2015/NSDUH-FFR2-2015.htm.

61. Ibid., https://www.samhsa.gov/data/sites/default/files/NSDUH-FFR2-2015/NSDUH-FFR2-2015.htm.

62. *Under the Counter,* 16.

63. Ibid., 14.

64. National Center on Addiction and Substance Abuse at Columbia University, Under the Counter: The Diversion and Abuse of Controlled Prescription Drugs in the U.S. (New York: Columbia University, 2005). CASA, 2005 49.

65. *Under the Counter.*

66. Ibid.

67. Jason A. Ford and Ryan D. Schroeder, "Academic Strain and Non-Medical Use of Prescription Stimulants among College Students," Deviant Behavior 30: 26–53. See Ford and Schroeder, 2008.

Chapter 1

1. Craig Reinarman and Harry G. Levine, eds., *Crack in America: Demon Drugs and Social Justice* (Berkeley: University of California Press, 1997).

2. Ibid.

3. "Epidemic Disease Occurrence," Centers for Disease Control and Prevention, https://www.cdc.gov/ophss/csels/dsepd/ss1978/lesson1/section11.html.

4. Holly Hedegaard, Margaret Warner, and Arialdi M. Minino, "Drug Overdose Deaths in the United States, 1999–2016," Centers for Disease Control and Prevention, https://www.cdc.gov/nchs/products/databriefs/db294.htm.

Chapter 2

1. Center for Behavioral Health Statistics and Quality, *2016 National Survey on Drug Use and Health: Detailed Tables* (Rockville, MD: Substance Abuse and Mental Health Services Administration, 2017).

2. Beth Han, Wilson M. Compton, Carlos Blanco, and Christopher M. Jones, "Correlate of Prescription Opioid Use: Misuse, Use Disorders, and Motivations for Misuse among US Adults," *Journal of Clinical Psychiatry* 79 (2018): e1–e11; Christopher M. Jones, Leonard J. Paulozzi, and Karin A. Mack, "Sources of Prescription Opioid Pain Relievers by Frequency of Past-Year Nonmedical Use: United States, 2008–2011," *JAMA Internal Medicine* 174 (2014): 802–803.

3. Richard Evans Schultes, Albert Hofmann, and Christian Rätsch, *Plants of the Gods: Their Sacred, Healing, and Hallucinogenic Powers* (Rochester, VT: Healing Arts, 2001), https://www.amazon.com/Plants-Gods-Sacred-Healing-Hallucinogenic/dp/0892819790.

4. Centers for Disease Control and Prevention, *Alcohol and Public Health: Alcohol-Related Disease Impact (ARDI); Average for United States 2006–2010 Alcohol-Attributable Deaths Due to Excessive Alcohol Use* (https://nccd.cdc.gov/DPH_ARDI/Default/Report.aspx?T=AAM&P=f6d7eda7-036e-4553-9968-9b17ffad620e&R=d7a9b303-48e9-4440-bf47-070a4827e1fd&M=8E1C5233-5640-4EE8-9247-1ECA7DA325B9&F=&D=).

5. Joseph R. Gusfeld, *Symbolic Crusade: Status Politics and the American Temperance Movement* (Chicago: University of Illinois Press, 1986).

6. Andrew Golub and Bruce D. Johnson, "Cohort Changes in Illegal Drug Use among Arrestees in Manhattan: From the Heroin Injection Generation to the Blunts Generation," *Substance Use and Misuse* 34 (1997): 1733–1763.

7. Carl D. Chambers, *An Assessment of Drug Use in the General Population* (Albany, NY: Narcotic Addiction Control Commission, 1971).

8. National Center on Addiction and Substance Abuse at Columbia University, *Under the Counter: The Diversion and Abuse of Controlled Prescription Drugs in the U.S.* (New York: Columbia University, 2005).

9. James A. Inciardi and Theodore J. Cicero, "Black Beauties, Gorilla Pills, Footballs, and Hillbilly Heroin: Some Reflection on Prescription Drug Abuse and Diversion Research over the Past 40 Years," *Journal of Drug Issues* 39 (2009): 101–114.

10. Sea Esteban McCabe, Brady T. West, and Carol J. Boyd, "Medical Use, Medical Misuse, and Nonmedical Use of Prescription Opioids: Results from a Longitudinal Study," *Pain* 154 (2013): 708–713.

11. Anna Lembke, *Drug Dealer, MD: How Doctors Were Duped, Patients Got Hooled, and Why It's So Hard to Stop* (Baltimore: Johns Hopkins University Press, 2016).

12. Russell K. Portenoy and Kathleen M. Foley, "Chronic Use of Opioid Analgesics in Non-Malignant Pain: Report of 38 Cases," *Pain* 25 (1986): 171–186.

13. Clifford R. Shaw and Henry D. McKay, *Juvenile Delinquency in Urban Areas* (Chicago: University of Chicago Press, 1942).

14. Jason A. Ford, Sarah Ann Sacra, and Alexis Yohros, "Neighborhood Characteristics and Prescription Drug Misuse among Adolescents: The Importance of Social Disorganization and Social Capital," *International Journal of Drug Policy* 4 (2017): 47–53.

15. Ronald Akers, *Deviant Behavior: A Social Learning Approach* (Belmont, CA: Wadsworth, 1985).

16. Edwin H. Sutherland, *Principles of Criminology* (Philadelphia: Lippincott, 1947).

17. Albert Bandura, *Social Learning Theory* (Englewood Cliffs, NJ: Prentice-Hall, 1977).

18. Jason A. Ford, "Social Learning Theory and Non-Medical Prescription Drug Use among Adolescents," *Sociological Spectrum* 28 (2008): 299–316; George E. Higgins, Margaret Mahoney, and Melissa L. Ricketts, "Nonsocial Reinforcement of the Nonmedical Use of Prescription Drugs: A Partial Test of Social Learning and Self-control Theories," *Journal of Drug Issues* 39 (2009): 949–964; Robert L. Peralta and Jennifer L. Steele, "Nonmedical Prescription Drug Use among US College Students at a Midwest University: A Partial Test of Social Learning Theory," *Substance Use and Misuse* 45 (2010): 865–887.

19. Travis Hirschi, *Causes of Delinquency* (Berkeley: University of California Press, 1969).

20. Jason A. Ford, "Non-Medical Prescription Drug Use among Adolescents: The Influence of Bonds to Family and School," *Youth & Society* 40 (2009): 336–352.

21. Michael R Gottfredson and Travis Hirschi, *A General Theory of Crime* (Stanford, CA: Stanford University Press, 1990).

22. Jason A. Ford and Lindsey Blumenstein, "Self-Control and Substance Use among College Students," *Journal of Drug Issues* 43(2013): 56–68.

23. Robert Agnew, "Foundation for a General Strain Theory of Delinquency," *Criminology* 30 (1992): 47–87.

24. Jason A. Ford and Ryan D. Schroeder, "Academic Strain and Non-Medical Use of Prescription Stimulants among College Students," *Deviant Behavior* 30 (2009): 26–53; Ryan D. Schroeder and Jason A. Ford, "Prescription Drug Misuse: A Test of Three Competing Criminological Theories," *Journal of Drug Issues* 42 (2012): 4–27.

25. Robert J. Sampson and John H. Laub, *Crime in the Making: Pathways and Turning Points through Life* (Boston: Harvard University Press, 1993).

26. Whitney D. Gunter, Steven P. Kurtz, Nicholas W. Bakken, and Daniel J. O'Connell, "Desisting from Prescription Drug Abuse: An Application of Growth Models to RX Opioid Users," *Journal of Drug Issues* 42(2012): 82–97.

27. Cindy Brooks Dollar and Bradley Ray, "Adult Nonmedical Prescription Drug Use: An Examination of Bond Theory," *Deviant Behavior* 34 (2013): 932–949; Cindy Brook Dollar and Joshua A. Hendrix, "The Importance of Romantic and Work Relations on Nonmedical Prescription Drug Use among Adults," *Sociological Spectrum* 35 (2015): 465–481.

28. Icek Ajzen, "From Intentions to Actions: a Theory of Planned Behavior," in *Action control: From Cognition to Behavior*, ed. J. Kuhl and J. Beckmann, 11–39 (New York: Springer, 1985).

29. Andre Gallucci, Ryan Martin, Alex Beaujean, and Stuart Usdan, "An Examination of the Misuse of Prescription Stimulants among College Students Using the Theory of Planned Behavior," *Psychology. Health, & Medicine* 20 (2015): 217–226.

30. Brian R. Flay and John Petraitis, "The Theory of Triadic Influence: A New Theory of Health Behavior with Implications for Preventive Interventions," in *Advances in Medical Sociology*, Vol. 4, *A Reconsideration of Models of Health Behavior Change*, ed. G. S. Albrecht, 19–44 (Greenwich, CT: JAI Press, 1994).

31. Niloofar Bavarian, Stephanie Sumstine, Sheena Cruz, Jocelyne Mendez, Cassandra Schroeder, and Summer Takeda, "Confirming the Prevalence, Characteristics, and Utility of Ecological Theory in Explaining Prescription Stimulant Misuse," *Journal of Drug Issues* 48 (2018): 118–113.

32. Jason A. Ford, Amy Reckdenwald, and Brianna Marquardt, "Prescription Drug Misuse and Gender," *Substance Use & Misuse* 49 (2014): 842–851.

33. Devin E. Banks, and Tamika C. Zapolski, "The Crossover Effect: A Review of Racial/Ethnic Variations in Risk for Substance Use and Substance Use Disorder across Development," *Current Addiction Reports* 5 (2018): 1–10.

34. Harvey L. Nicholson and Jason A. Ford, "Correlates of Prescription Opioid Misuse among Black Adults: Findings from the 2015 National Survey on Drug Use and Health," *Drug and Alcohol Dependence* 18 (2018): 264–267; Jason A. Ford and Khary K. Rigg, "Racial/Ethnic Differences in Factors That Place Adolescents at Risk for Prescription Opioid Misuse," *Prevention Science* 1 (2015): 633–641.

35. John M. Wallace Jr., "Explaining Race Differences in Adolescent and Young Adult Drug Use: The Role of Racialized Social Systems," *Drugs & Society* 14 (1998): 21–36.

36. Katherine M. Keyes, Magdalena Cerda, Joanne E. Brady, Jennifer R. Havens, and Sandro Galea, "Understanding the Rural-Urban Differences in Nonmedical Prescription Opioid Use and Abuse in the United States," *American Journal of Public Health* 104 (2014): e52–e59.

37. William C. Becker, David A. Fiellin, Joseph O. Merrill, and Susan H. Busch, "Opioid Use Disorder in the United States: Insurance Status and Treatment Access," *Drug and Alcohol Dependence* 94 (2008): 207–213.

38. Alexander S. Perlmutter, Sarah C. Conner, Mirko Savone, June H. Kim, Luis E. Segura, and Silvia S. Martins, "Is Employment Status in Adults over 25 Years Old Associated with Nonmedical Prescription Opioid and Stimulant Use?," *Social Psychiatry and Psychiatric Epidemiology* 52 (2017): 291–298.

39. Arthur Hughes, Matthew R. Williams, Rachel N. Lipari, Jonaki Bose, Elizabeth A. P. Copello, and Larry A. Kroutil, *Prescription Drug Use and Misuse in the United States: Results from the 2015 National Survey on Drug Use and Health* (Washington, DC: Substance Abuse and Mental Health Services Administration, 2015).

40. Han et al., "Correlate of Prescription Opioid Use."

41. Rachel N. Lipari and Arthur Hughes, *How People Obtain the Prescription Pain Relievers They Misuse*, The CBHSQ Report, January 12 (Rockville, MD: Center for Behavioral Health Statistics and Quality, Substance Abuse and Mental Health Services Administration, 2017).

42. Jones, Paulozzi, and Mack, "Sources of Prescription Opioid Pain Relievers by Frequency of Past-Year Nonmedical Use."

43. Andrew Golub, Bruce D. Johnson, and Eloise Dunlap, "Subcultural Evolution and Illicit Drug Use," *Addiction Research and Theory* 13 (2005): 217–229.

44. Golub and Johnson, "Cohort Changes in Illegal Drug Use among Arrestees in Manhattan."

45. Norman Zinberg, *Drug, Set, and Setting: The Basis for Controlled Intoxicant Use* (New Haven, CT: Yale, 1986).

46. Golub and Johnson, "Cohort Changes in Illegal Drug Use among Arrestees in Manhattan."

47. Talcott Parsons, *The Social System* (Glencoe, IL: Free Press, 1951).

Chapter 3

1. German Lopes, "When a Drug Epidemic's Victims Are White: How Racial Bias and Segregation Molded a Gentler Rhetorical Response to the Opioid Crisis," Vox, April 4, 2017, https://www.vox.com/identities/2017/4/4/15098746/opioid-heroin-epidemic-race.

2. Jessica Ravitz, "Inside the Secret Lives of Functioning Heroin Addicts," CNN, February 27, 2018, https://www.cnn.com/2018/02/27/health/functioning-heroin-addicts/index.html.

3. Wilson M. Compton, Christopher M. Jones, and Grant T. Baldwin, "Relationship between Nonmedical Prescription-Opioid Use and Heroin Use," *New England Journal of Medicine* 374 (2016): 154–163.

4. Theodore J. Cicero et al., "The Changing Face of Heroin Use in the United States: A Retrospective Analysis of the Past 50 Years," *JAMA Psychiatry* 71 (2014): 821–826.

5. Christopher M. Jones, "Heroin Use and Heroin Use Risk Behaviors among Nonmedical Users of Prescription Opioid Pain Relievers—United States, 2002–2004 and 2008–2010," *Drug and Alcohol Dependence* 132 (2013): 95–100.

6. Compton, Jones, and Baldwin, "Relationship between Nonmedical Prescription-Opioid Use and Heroin Use," 160.

7. Jones, "Heroin Use and Heroin Use Risk Behaviors among Nonmedical Users of Prescription Opioid Pain Relievers," 98.

8. *2011 Heroin Domestic Monitoring Program: Drug Intelligence Report* (Washington, DC: U.S. Department of Justice, Drug Enforcement Administration, 2013).

9. Ibid.

10. *National Heroin Threat Assessment Summary—Updated* (Washington, DC: U.S. Department of Justice, Drug Enforcement Administration, 2016).

11. Anne Case and Angus Denton, "Rising Morbidity and Mortality in Midlife among White Non-Hispanic Americans in the 21st Century," *Proceedings of the National Academy of Sciences of the United States of America* 112 (2015): 1581.

Chapter 4

1. S. M. Fishman, J. S. Papazian, S. Gonzalez, P. S. Riches, and A. Gilson, "Regulating Opioid Prescribing through Prescription Monitoring Programs: Balancing Drug Diversion and Treatment of Pain," *Pain Medicine* 5 (2004): 309–324.

2. J. Worley, "Prescription Drug Monitoring Programs, a Response to Doctor Shopping: Purpose, Effectiveness, and Directions for Future Research," *Issues in Mental Health Nursing* 33 (2012): 319–328.

3. Fishman et al., "Regulating Opioid Prescribing through Prescription Monitoring Programs"; Worley, "Prescription Drug Monitoring Programs, a Response to Doctor Shopping."

4. L. N. Sacco, J. H. Duff, and A. K. Sarata, *Prescription Drug Monitoring Programs* (Washington, DC: Congressional Research Service, 2018).

5. Ibid.

6. M. M. Ali, W. N. Dowd, T. Classen, R. Mutter, and S. P. Novak, "Prescription Drug Monitoring Programs, Nonmedical Use of Prescription Drugs, and Heroin Use: Evidence from the National Survey of Drug Use and Health," *Addictive Behaviors* 69 (2017): 65–77.

7. *Research to Address the Opioid Crisis: Approaches to Data Linkage* (Washington, DC: Department of Health and Human Services, 2017).

8. U.S. Department of Health and Human Services, Substance Abuse and Mental Health Services Administration, Results from the 2016 National Survey on Drug Use and Health: Summary of National Findings, September 2017, https://www.samhsa.gov/ data/sites/default/files/NSDUH-FFR1-2016/NSDUH-FFR1-2016.htm (hereinafter: 2016 National Survey on Drug Use and Health). Department of Health and Human Services & Assistant Secretary for Planning and Evaluation, 2016.

9. Fishman et al., "Regulating Opioid Prescribing through Prescription Monitoring Programs."

10. Ibid.; Sacco, Duff, and Sarata, *Prescription Drug Monitoring Programs.*

11. A. M. Gilson, S. M. Fishman, B. L. Wilsey, C. Casamalhuapa, and H. Baxi, "Time Series Analysis of California's Prescription Drug Monitoring Program: Impact on Prescribing and Multiple Provider Episodes," *Journal of Pain* 13 (2012): 103–111.

12. Fishman et al., "Regulating Opioid Prescribing through Prescription Monitoring Programs."

13. Ali et al., "Prescription Drug Monitoring Programs, Nonmedical Use of Prescription Drugs, and Heroin Use."

14. Ibid.; P. Moyo, L. Simoni-Wastila, B. A. Griffin, E. Onukwugha, D. Harrington, G. C. Alexander, and F. Palumbo, "Impact of Prescribing Drug

Monitoring Programs (PDMPs) on Opioid Utilization among Medicare Beneficiaries in 10 States," *Addiction* 112 (2017): 1784–1796.

15. N. M. Perez, W. G. Jennings, Y. Wange, and C. Delcher, "Law Enforcement Officers' Perceptions of Florida's Prescription Drug Monitoring Program," *Journal of Contemporary Criminal Justice* 33 (2017): 368–379.

16. L. Rutkow, K. C. Smith, A. Y. Lai, J. S. Vernick, C. S. Davis, and G. C. Alexander, "Prescription Drug Monitoring Program Design and Function: A Qualitative Analysis," *Drug and Alcohol Dependence* 180 (2017): 395–400; N. J. Pauly, S. Slavova, C. Delcher, P. R. Freeman, and J. Talbert, "Features of Prescription Drug Monitoring Programs Associated with Reduced Rates of Prescription Opioid-related Poisonings," *Drug and Alcohol Dependence* 184 (2018): 26–32.

17. Pauly et al., "Features of Prescription Drug Monitoring Programs Associated with Reduced Rates of Prescription Opioid-related Poisonings."

18. Sacco, Duff, and Sarata, *Prescription Drug Monitoring Programs.*

19. Rutkow et al., "Prescription Drug Monitoring Program Design and Function."

20. Pauly et al., "Features of Prescription Drug Monitoring Programs Associated with Reduced Rates of Prescription Opioid-related Poisonings."

21. Ibid.

22. Worley, "Prescription Drug Monitoring Programs, a Response to Doctor Shopping."

23. H. Matusow, A. Rosenblum, and M. Parrino, "Prescription Drug Monitoring Program Utilization among 15 Opioid Treatment Programs," *Journal of Substance Abuse Treatment* 85 (2018): 17–20.

24. Ali et al., "Prescription Drug Monitoring Programs, Nonmedical Use of Prescription Drugs, and Heroin Use."

25. Pauly et al., "Features of Prescription Drug Monitoring Programs Associated with Reduced Rates of Prescription Opioid-related Poisonings."

26. J. C. Veilleux, P. J. Colvin, J. Anderson, C. York, and A. Heinz, "A Review of Opioid Dependence Treatment: Pharmacological and Psychosocial Interventions to Treat Opioid Addiction," *Clinical Psychology Review* 30 (2010): 155–166.

27. Ibid.

28. T. S. Shippenberg, V. I. Chefer, and A. C. Thompson, "Delta-Opioid Receptor Antagonists Prevent Sensitization to the Conditioned Rewarding Effects of Morphine," *Biological Psychiatry* 65 (2009): 169–174; Veilleux et al., "A Review of Opioid Dependence Treatment"; Shippenberg, Chefer, and Thompson, "Delta-Opioid Receptor Antagonists Prevent Sensitization to the Conditioned Rewarding Effects of Morphine."

29. Veilleux et al., "A Review of Opioid Dependence Treatment."

30. Shippenberg, Chefer, and Thompson, "Delta-Opioid Receptor Antagonists Prevent Sensitization to the Conditioned Rewarding Effects of Morphine."

31. *Principles of Drug Addiction Treatment: A Research Based Guide*, The National Institute of Drug Addiction, https://www.drugabuse.gov/publications/principles-drug-addiction-treatment-research-based-guide-third-edition/principles-effective-treatment.

32. L. Amato, S. Minozzi, M. Davoli, S. Vecchi, M. M. Ferri, and S. Mayet, "Psychosocial and Pharmacological Treatments versus Pharmacological Treatments for Opioid Detoxification," Cochran Database of Systematic Reviews, https://www.cochrane.org/CD005031/ADDICTN_psychosocial-and-pharmacological-treatments-versus-pharmacological-treatments-for-opioid-detoxification.

33. M. Pugatch, J. R. Knight, P. McGuiness, L. Sherritt, and S. Levy, "A Group Therapy Program for Opioid-Dependent Adolescents and Their Parents," *Substance Abuse* 35 (2014): 435–441.

34. M. Hasanovic, A. Kuldija, I. Pajevic, A. Delic, A. Sutovic, and D. Stanisic, "Medical Assisted Treatment of Opiate Dependence with Buprenorphine/Naloxone (Suboxone) or Heroin Addicts in Prison Who Are Aging Penalties," *European Psychiatry* 27 (2012): 1–1.

35. Ibid.

36. Ibid.

37. E. Dyb, "Housing First or No Housing? Housing and Homelessness at the End of the Alcohol and Drug Treatment," *International Journal on Drug Policy* 36 (2016): 76–84.

38. C. Barrowclough, G. Haddock, R. Beardmore, P. Conrod, T. Craig, L. Davies, and T. Wykes, "Evaluating Integrated MI and CBT for People with Psychosis and Substance Misuse: Recruitment, Retention, and Sample Characteristics of MIDAS Trial," *Addictive Behaviors* 34 (2009): 859–866.

39. C. Drummond, C. Kouimtsidis, M. Reynolds, I. Russell, C. Godfrey, M. McCusker, and S. Porter, "The Effectiveness and Cost Effectiveness of Cognitive Behavior Therapy for Opiate Misusers in Methadone Maintenance Treatment: A Multicenter, Randomized, Controlled Trial," *Drugs: Education, Prevention, & Policy* 12 (2005): 69–76; J. Morgenstern, K. A. Blanchard, T. J. Morgan, E. Labouvie, and J. Hayaki, "Testing the Effectiveness of Cognitive-Behavioral Treatment for Substance Abuse in a Community Setting: Within Treatment and Posttreatment Findings," *Journal of Consulting and Clinical Psychology* 69 (2001): 1007–1017; J. S. Beck, *Cognitive Therapy: Basics and Beyond*, 2nd ed. (New York: Guilford, 2011).

40. C. C. DiClemente, "Motivation for Change: Implications for Substance Abuse Treatment," *Psychological Science* 10 (1999): 209–213.

41. M. Magill and L. A. Ray, "Cognitive-Behavioral Treatment with Adult Alcohol and Illicit Drug Users: A Meta-Analysis of Randomized Controlled Trials." *Journal of Studies on Alcohol and Drugs* 70 (2009): 516–527.

42. DiClemente, "Motivation for Change: Implications for Substance Abuse Treatment."

43. Ibid.

44. E. L. Deci and R. M. Ryan, *Intrinsic Motivation and Self-Determination in Human Behavior* (New York: Plenum, 1985).

45. N. M. Petry and B. Martin, "Low-Cost Contingency Management for Treating Cocaine- and Opioid-Abusing Methadone Patients," *Journal of Consulting and Clinical Psychology* 73 (2002): 354–359.

46. T. S. Ainscough, A. McNeill, J. Strang, R. Calder, and L. S. Brose, "Contingency Management Interventions for Non-Prescribed Drug Use during

Treatment for Opiate Addiction: A Systematic Review and Meta-Analysis," *Drug and Alcohol Dependence* 178 (2017): 318–339.

47. Ibid.

48. C. S. Sayegh, S. J. Huey, E. J. Zara, and K. Jhaveri, "Follow-Up Treatment Effects of Contingency Management and Motivational Interviewing on Substance Use: A Meta-Analysis," *Psychology of Addictive Behaviors* 31 (2017): 403–414.

49. P. G. Barnett, J. H. Rodgers, and D. A. Bloch, "A Meta-Analysis Comparing Buprenorphine to Methadone for Treatment of Opiate Dependence," *Addiction* 96 (2002): 683–690.

50. Ibid.

51. B. K. Zedler et al., "Buprenorphine Compared with Methadone to Treat Pregnant Women with Opioid Use Disorder: A Systematic Review and Meta-Analysis of Safety in the Mother, Fetus and Child," *Addiction* 111 (2016): 2131–2133.

52. A. T. McCellan and A. M. Woodworth, "The Affordable Care Act and Treatment for 'Substance Use Disorders': Implications of Ending Segregated Behavioral Healthcare," *Journal of Substance Abuse Treatment* 46 (2014): 541–545.

53. Ibid.

54. "Analysis: Most Short-Term Health Plans Don't Cover Drug Treatment for Prescription Drugs, and None Cover Maternity Care," Henry Kaiser Foundation, April 23, 2018, https://www.kff.org/health-reform/press-release/analysis-most-short-term-health-plans-dont-cover-drug-treatment-or-prescription-drugs-and-none-cover-maternity-care/.

55. Ibid.

56. Ibid.

57. Ibid.

58. Ibid.

59. Ibid.

60. Ibid.

61. Ibid.

62. Ibid.

63. E. Winstanley, C. M. Wilder, and A. K. Clark, "A Systematic Review of Community Opioid Overdose Prevention and Naloxone Distribution Programs," *Journal of Addiction Medicine* 8 (2014): 153–163.

64. D. Kerr, P. Dietze, and A. M. Kelly, "Intranasal Naloxone for the Treatment of Suspected Heroin Overdose," *Addiction* 103 (2008): 379–386.

65. T. C. Green, R. Heimer, and L. E. Grau, "Distinguishing Signs of Opioid Overdose and Indication for Naloxone: An Evaluation of Six Overdose Training and Naloxone Distribution Programs in the United States," *Addiction* 103 (2008): 979–989.

66. Winstanley, Wilder, and Clark, "A Systematic Review of Community Opioid Overdose Prevention and Naloxone Distribution Programs."

67. C. Rowe, G. M. Santos, E. Vittinghoff, E. Wheeler, P. Davidson, and P. O. Coffin, "Predictors of Participant Engagement and Naloxone Utilization in a

Community-Based Naloxone Distribution Program," *Addiction* 110 (2015): 1301–1310; Kerr, Dietze, and Kelly, "Intranasal Naloxone for the Treatment of Suspected Heroin Overdose."

68. R. E. Cash, J. Kinsman, R. P. Crowe, M. K. Rivard, M. Faul, and A. R. Panchal, "Naloxone Administration Frequency during Emergency Medical Service Events—United States, 2012–2016," *MMWR Morb Mortal Wkly Rep* 67 (2018): 850–853.

Chapter 5

1. Charles E. Menifield, Winfield H. Rose, John Homa, and Anita Brewer Cunningham, "The Media's Portrayal of Urban and Rural School Violence: A Preliminary Analysis," *Deviant Behavior* 22 (2001): 447–464.

2. Ibid., 450.

3. S. Patrick Kachur et al., "School-Associated Violent Deaths in the United States, 1992 to 1994," *JAMA* 275 (1996): 1729–1733.

4. *Annual Report on School Safety* (Washington, DC: U.S. Department of Education and U.S. Department of Justice, 1998).

5. Shanto Iyengar and Donald R. Kinder, *News That Matters: Television and American Opinion* (Chicago: University of Chicago Press, 1987), 33.

6. Shanto Iyengar, *Is Anyone Responsible? How Television Frames Political Issues* (Chicago: University of Chicago Press, 1991), 125.

7. Daniel Patrick Moynihan, "Defining Deviancy Down: How We've Become Accustomed to Alarming Levels of Crime and Destructive Behavior," *American Educator* (1993): 10–18.

8. Menifield et al., "The Media's Portrayal of Urban and Rural School Violence," 461–462.

9. James S. Goodwin, Yong-Fang Kuo, David Brown, David Juurlink, and Mukaita Raji, "Association of Chronic Opioid Use with Presidential Voting Patterns in U.S. Counties in 2016," *JAMA Network Open* 1 (2018): 1–11.

10. William Chambliss, *Crime and the Legal Process* (New York: McGraw-Hill, 1969).

11. "The War on Marijuana in Black and White: Billions of Dollars Wasted on Racially Biased Arrests," American Civil Liberties Union, June 2013, https://www.aclu.org/files/assets/aclu-thewaronmarijuana-rel2.pdf.

12. Richard Quinney, *Critique of Legal Order: Crime Control in Capitalist Society* (New Brunswick, NJ: Transaction Publishers, 1974).

13. Craig Reinarman and Harry G. Levine, eds., *Crack in America: Demon Drugs and Social Justice* (Berkeley: University of California Press, 1997).

14. Ibid.

15. Holly Hedegaard, Margaret Warner, and Arialdi M. Minino, "Drug Overdose Deaths in the United States, 1999–2016," Centers for Disease Control and Prevention, 2017, https://www.cdc.gov/nchs/products/databriefs/db294.htm.

16. "Vital Statistics Rapid Release: Provisional Drug Overdose Death Counts," Centers for Disease Control and Prevention, 2018, https://www.cdc.gov/nchs/nvss/vsrr/drug-overdose-data.htm.

17. Michael Martinez, Ana Cabrera, and Sara Weisfeldt, "Denver Mom Survives Darkness of Prescription Drug Abuse Epidemic," CNN, July 23, 2014, https://www-m.cnn.com/2014/07/23/us/prescription-drug-heroin-abuse-epidemic/index.html?r=https%3A%2F%2Fwww.google.com%2F.

18. Colin Moynihan, "Don't Call Her a Victim: After Surviving Opioids, Nan Goldin Goes after the Makers," *New York Times*, January 22, 2018, https://www.nytimes.com/2018/01/22/arts/design/nan-goldin-oxycontin-addiction-opioid.html.

19. Alan Bavley, "Prescription Pills, Addiction 'Hell': Rachelle Allen's Story of Opioid Abuse Offers Look inside U.S. Epidemic," *Kansas City Star*, February 27, 2016, https://www.kansascity.com/living/health-fitness/article62909822.html.

20. Margot Sanger-Katz, "Bleak New Estimates in Drug Epidemic: A Record 72,000 Overdose Deaths in 2017," *New York Times*, August 15, 2018, https://www.nytimes.com/2018/08/15/upshot/opioids-overdose-deaths-rising-fentanyl.html.

21. Fallon Glick, "New CDC Report Says Needle Exchange in Scott County, Indiana, Is Working," WDRB, March 7, 2018, http://www.wdrb.com/story/37674122/new-cdc-report-says-needle-exchange-in-scott-county-indiana-is-working.

22. Keridwen Cornelius, "Sewage Is Helping Cities Flush Out the Opioid Crisis: Poop Studies Are Helping Communities Make Intervention Decisions," *Scientific American*, May 25, 2018, https://www.scientificamerican.com/article/sewage-is-helping-cities-flush-out-the-opioid-crisis/.

23. Melvin D. Livingston, Tracey E. Barnett, Chris Delcher, and Alexander C. Wagenaar, "Recreational Cannabis Legalization and Opioid-Related Deaths in Colorado, 2000–2015," *American Journal of Public Health* 107 (2017): 1827–1829.

Index

About the Authors

Ryan D. Schroeder is a professor and the department chair in the Department of Sociology at the University of Louisville. He has published dozens of journal articles and book chapters addressing crime and deviance, with a specific focus on issues related to drug use, families, and religion. In 2009, Schroeder received the James F. Short Outstanding Article Award from the Crime, Law, and Deviance section of the American Sociological Association for an essay published in the *American Journal of Sociology*.

Jason A. Ford is an associate professor of sociology at the University of Central Florida. His research focuses on substance use, particularly prescription drug misuse, among adolescents and young adults. Ford's primary interests lie within the field of criminology, where he examines theoretical explanations of misuse and assesses the relationship between misuse and offending behavior. His secondary interests lie within the field of medical sociology, where his work examines social determinants of drug use/misuse, including age, gender, race/ethnicity, education, sports involvement, and religiosity. Much of his published work utilizes data from the National Survey on Drug Use and Health, a leading source of epidemiological data on substance use in the United States.

George E. Higgins is a professor in the Department of Criminal Justice at the University of Louisville. He received his PhD in criminology from Indiana University of Pennsylvania in 2001 and is the current editor of the *Journal of Criminal Justice Education*. Higgins's most recent publications appear or are forthcoming in the *Journal of Criminal Justice, Criminal Justice and Behavior, Justice Quarterly, Deviant Behavior,* and *Youth and Society.*

www.ingramcontent.com/pod-product-compliance
Ingram Content Group UK Ltd.
Pitfield, Milton Keynes, MK11 3LW, UK
UKHW020807290926
15470UKWH00003B/1013

9 781440 85769